# THE LAWS OF

# STRENGTH

CONOR O'FLYNN

*The Laws of Strength*

This book is dedicated to those looking to live big.

This book is also dedicated to my family. I've been left a heritage of writing and doing things our own way. As it turns out, I have some sense of practicality, too. A nice blend for bookbuilding.

Many thanks to my various clientele: you have all inspired me to write this book in one way or another.

Lastly, this book is dedicated to the memory of my dog Dexter. Dexter was so much more than a dog to me. He was my own personal coach throughout the writing of this book.

*The Laws of Strength*

*The Laws of Strength*

# PREFACE

This book is the product of experience in life and in practice. The foundations for the book were laid in my preteen years. In those years, I learned the value of being strong and my ability to influence my strength. I've been working on becoming stronger ever since.

The Laws of Strength needed to be written. The idea came from varied experiences I've had with patients and clients alike. Too many patients were in pain because they lacked basic structural integrity. Others were in pain because they lacked the willpower to use that integrity properly. Too many clients were strong in specific ways, but not resilient as a whole.

In an effort to avoid repeating myself in the clinic and gym, I started writing blog articles. The messages are getting through, but some of the messages deserve more legitimacy and permanence.

The Laws of Strength implores you to improve yourself through strength training. Aging becomes a legitimate concern early in our lives. Despite ever evolving medical practices and technology, most people will start aching, feeling older, moving slower and cutting things from their lives at an early age. Not only is this unnecessary, it is the wrong way to go about increasing your chronological age.

Through strength training, you can become more resilient,

capable and happy. Even for the younger folk reading this, the foundations you lay now can help you or hurt you long term: there is no time like the present. The real impetus to start this book came from observing younger people in the gym: most have no idea what they're doing, but they sure think that they do.

There aren't enough therapists recommending serious strength training to patients. The practice is treated as though it is controversial or dangerous, but this is untrue when you perform as detailed in this book. More trainers need to remove their heads from their asses and take their practice seriously.

As professionals in various health and fitness related fields, we need to push strength. We need to teach the value of strength, and the value in the pursuit of strength. The human body is a magnificent gift: this book is an effort to teach you how to honour and improve on that gift.

*The Laws of Strength*

*The Laws of Strength*

# THE CONQUEST

The Conquest methods are a challenge, a call to action, and a way of life simultaneously.

We, of the modern world, are lucky enough to be challenged by problems that didn't exist for our predecessors. Trace your lineage back just a few generations and you'll see that your forebears were challenged as much by the external environment as they were by their own internal environment. They would succeed and fail at things, but the intention to succeed and work hard was present out of necessity. Failure could come from a lack of resources and unforgiving surroundings.

In the Information Age, our problems are illustrated by battery life and text-neck. We have greater abundance in all of the factors necessary for life, and we don't make good use of them. We're surrounded by time and effort saving technologies, but we use our newfound free time to enjoy the technology more. Enjoying life certainly isn't a bad thing. Enjoying technology isn't inherently bad. However, many of our choices to seek out pleasure and comfort are leading us toward a precipice.

The Conquest way is not the path of least resistance. It is the most efficient path to becoming able to handle anything. It is the most efficient way to become a strong, self-sufficient human being. We don't hide from resistance, and we don't glorify hard work that is applied in a foolish direction.

The path that allows you to be happy, healthy and move towards actualization exists, but this path is full of resistance. Rather than avoid the path because you'll need to fight your way through it, learn to love the fight. Engage in something challenging that strengthens you. Encounter difficulty and know that the solution will bring you new strength to help yourself and others.

The Conquest way is not a lifting program, a diet or a self-help book. This is a way of life based around learning, applying effort, and continually growing. This is a call to return to a way of life that allowed our ancestors to progress and build a better future for us. This is a call to improve on their mistakes and advance with our advancing technology.

This book was written for those that need to understand resistance training. It's written for the experienced trainee and the complete novice alike. In short, it is written for anyone that wants to make continual progress. It is written for those unhappy with the declining physical in their lives. It is written for those that want more.

Life is growth. If you aren't growing, you aren't living. Learn to continue your growth as a trainee and a person. The life of the student is one of humility, purposeful work and meaning. The life of the student is also one of difficulty and resistance. Living a fulfilling and purposeful life comes at a cost.

There is no better analogy for this relationship than resistance training. You can take a frame riddled with frailties and make it stronger.

Through the methodical application of resistance and effort this frailty becomes strength. It is no coincidence that this process also strengthens the mind. The will to act, the desire to become greater, and the ability to live your own life to its greatest potential all come from engaging resistance.

Choose to live your life. Choose to encounter resistance and difficulty on your own terms. Choose to grow from your effort. In the process of applying resistance, you'll learn a lot about yourself and others. You'll learn to grow as a person, and you'll learn to help others grow as well.

Our forebears left us a heritage of strength and perseverance. It is time we remember and honour that heritage with work of our own.

Choose your challenges. Engage the resistance. Grow. Progress. Work. Live. Enjoy.

*The Laws of Strength*

# CHAPTER I

# WHY LIFT?

This is a book about strength. In today's world, I'm writing about a rare and valuable trait that few possess but everyone needs. If you're reading this, you may fear that you need to be stronger. You're probably right.

The practice of lifting weighted objects is ancient. We see evidence of feats of strength in art and historical records. We're aware that most cultures held competitions featuring exhibitions and celebrations of strength. These competitions and practices are contrived efforts; the efforts aren't directly vital to human survival.

Strength is.

Long before we competed or celebrated with our physical strength, it was an absolutely essential asset for survival. Life was simpler for early human beings; it essentially came down to making as many children as possible before you were killed by a large predator or starved to death. For the most part we no longer face such predatory challenges in the developed world.

When you look back far enough, you realize that humanity is built on a solid foundation of physical capability. Without learning to walk on two feet, we would never have become proficient at using tools such as spears and twitter. Without the need for tools, we wouldn't have developed opposable thumbs. Without opposable thumbs, we wouldn't have been able to advance the complexity of our tools and our movement patterns. **Most importantly, without these physical advancements, our brains would never have developed enough for us to pursue better tomorrows.**

Our brain outpaced the cranial development of other creatures largely because we could perform tasks with greater complexity. The only way you can perform tasks with any complexity is to have a base of strength that allows you to do so. I fear that our modern craniums may begin to shrink again over time. Thanks Netflix.

Imagine an ancient-era version of yourself. I bet you immediately envisioned someone more robust than you are now. Pursued by predators, hungry all the time, needing to provide for a family and tribe. You'd better be robust, you've got work to do.

Ancient you is probably cold, because you're obviously wearing a Flintstones-cartoon-esque-toga. Do you have the option to refuse the hunt because you're tired? Can you tell your tribe-mates to do the work because your spear is too heavy? Who the hell is going to cart your kids around from site to site? Here's a shocker: you don't have a chair to sit on.

We come from a universal heritage of strong people. These people may not have lived long, but they lived a lot longer than soft modern humans would if we were placed in the same environment. They may not have had as many twitter followers, but they would literally walk across a continent to feed their families. Many modern people won't get out of their chairs to go to the kitchen.

Our modern world is a gift. Many great people contributed to the innovations that we should be thankful for. That said, we can't forget our heritage. We're in tremendous danger of growing weak as a society. If that doesn't scare you, read on. You'll quickly learn that a lack of strength can be the primary factor leading to pain, depression, disease and death before your time.

This book is about erasing those possibilities from your future.

*The Laws of Strength*

# MYTHS, GIFTS AND WHYS

Sometimes I think I'm living in some bizarre twilight zone. It's bizarre to me that not everyone performs some form of strength training AT LEAST weekly. Considering that we need strength on a daily basis, it makes sense to work on building strength frequently.

Not everyone performs formal exercise. If this is you, read these next few paragraphs very carefully. Everyone needs to exercise. Everyone. Every-one. It doesn't matter if you sit at a desk for a living, if you're recently retired, or you're a young stud that performs physical work every day. Everyone needs formal exercise.

You may not need to go to the gym. We'll get into that later. However, you need a formal exercise intervention for several reasons. Dip into your heritage again and you'll see why. Go back just one or two generations and look at how life has changed. We don't need to move for anything now. As of this writing, you can literally get any food or booze you want delivered to your door. You can have access to endless digital content from any one of ten devices you own. You can see friends over skype. You can work online. Life has never been less physical than it is today.

Yet there is a prevalent belief that we get the activity we need throughout the day. No, you don't. Your grandparents probably did in the first half of the 20th century. Their parents definitely did. Getting your 10,000 steps is great, but it only scratches the surface. If you're under the impression that simply comporting yourself to your car a few dozen times and 'taking the stairs' covers your fitness bases, you'd best leave that belief behind.

Our desire for physical comfort typically takes priority over our need for strength. The irony in this relationship is that weakness will always lead you to physical discomfort eventually. Leave behind the idea that your body is used the same way as the typical 19th century factory worker or farmer. You aren't that person, and that life doesn't exist anymore in the modern world.

So if your daily incidental activity doesn't cover your bases, does getting your 10,000 steps fit the bill? Not a chance. Walking a certain number of steps is a great goal to have every day, but it only makes you good at taking steps on a level surface. There is no overload on your tissues by achieving your daily requirement. It won't make you strong enough to climb stairs without pain. It won't allow you to run for the bus or plane. It won't allow you to lift and carry your kids or grandkids. I fear our weakness will continue to grow in the delusion of the walking/pedometer age.

Of the arbitrary number of steps you take every day, how many of them really challenge you? At what number do you think, "Man, I don't know if I can take another step without collapsing"? I'm betting that you *never* get to that point. This is a safe bet, because you've stacked the cards in your favour.

Walking is low impact. Walking is low load. Walking is low intensity by definition, otherwise it would become running. Walking is accomplished by placing a significant amount of loading on the bones, joints and connective tissues; passive tissues that allow us to evade our lack of strength.

There isn't much chance of overload, unless you are in fact 13 months old. For you to reach overload, you'ld probably need to walk until your feet were covered in blisters. At this point it is probably the blisters stopping you, not muscular fatigue. Even if walking or carrying groceries did produce overload, it would be a miniscule tiny. Any adaptation from these activities would be insignificant; it wouldn't help you with your other physical needs.

There is nothing wrong with getting groceries, or with accumulating steps every day. There is something wrong with assuming that this covers your bases. This blindness is the best way to ensure that you age quickly and thoroughly. As none of us want to age, I would assume that most people would be open to a better solution.

Resistance training is a must. There are endless reasons. In ten minutes per day, you can train the muscles harder than you can with 10,000 steps. You can train them more specifically: to reduce back pain, to allow you to play rec sports or hike, or to look better on the beach. You can accomplish a lot with ten hard, dedicated minutes. You can accomplish even more with 20 minutes.

Get over your fears or hesitations about resistance training. The same irrational questions that plagued the resistance training world 30 years ago are still prevalent today. Let's go through a couple of myths to give you a clearer picture of reality.

*The Laws of Strength*

# MYTH: RESISTANCE TRAINING IS DANGEROUS.

Not even close. Running is actually the most injurious recreational activity. If we count resistance training as a recreational sport, it is actually safer than all other rec sports. Controlled, appropriately loaded movements are not only safe, they're protective. Consider this; loading your entire body with a perfectly performed deadlift disperses the load well and makes you stronger. Lifting your groceries with no lifting skill can herniate a disc, making you considerably weaker.

If you never learn to deadlift, eventually you'll try to pick something up off the ground or pull on a sock and you'll herniate a disc in your lower back. Why? You didn't know how to disperse the load. Your tissues weren't prepared for the load. The effort you put into this meager task was more concentrated on fragile, passive tissues than a well-performed heavy deadlift. Not only is lifting safe, it actually makes life safer.

Strength training teaches you to use more muscle and technique in daily life. Getting good at lifting inherently helps you avoid chronic joint stress and pain.

## MYTH: RESISTANCE TRAINING REQUIRES YOU TO LIFT 'WEIGHTS'.

This may be the greatest lifting myth of all. Resistance training means that your tissues are encountering resistance, period. This doesn't describe where the resistance comes from, or how you're using it.

Here's a shocker: gravity is resistance. It may not be much - depending on how much you weigh - but it is exerting a force on you that must be countered with muscular force (or terrible posture). If you've ever stood up from a chair, you've performed some resistance training. Ha! You're a convert already!

If you take a step - one of your 10,000 per day - you experience forces between two and four times your bodyweight every time your foot hits the ground. Without resisting that force, you'd crumble to the ground on every step. When running, you'll see forces between five and seven times bodyweight. When jumping, that number can reach over 10x bodyweight.

If you decide to play ultimate frisbee or you run to answer the phone and have to dodge your furniture, you're sprinting and rapidly changing directions multiple times. The forces acting on your joints in these situations are *massive*. These maximal or near maximal exertions create a chaotic environment. The movement is so complex that the joints encounter serious risk.

Performing a simple bodyweight squat means lifting *just* your bodyweight. You can learn to control the joint actions to ensure safety. The environment is closed and controllable. If this is too easy for you, you can do a split squat, which uses your bodyweight to pick on one leg at a time. If this is still too easy, you can start learning single-leg exercises.

In each of these scenarios, the resistance forces come from your bodyweight. You manipulate the movement to change the resistance. Ergo, having bodyweight means that you can and do resistance training already. You'd better learn how to do it properly.

If we add simple implements like a jug of water, a dumbbell, kettlebell, or a light resistance band, I can give you a dozen different workouts that will be challenging for quite some time. If you don't choose your challenges, you'll be challenged in ways you didn't choose.

# MYTH: KIDS AND THE ELDERLY SHOULDN'T LIFT WEIGHTS.

Wrong. So, so wrong. The evil of aging is illustrated well in the dramatic decrease of physical capacity over time. Resistance training increases physical capacity. It's actually possible to get stronger at any age, and doing so will make you less likely to fall or otherwise hurt yourself. This has been thoroughly researched, with study participants in their 90's showing strength increases leading to a lower incidence of falls. At a certain point in your life, falls will become your primary health concern...or maybe they already are!

Lifting weights also strengthens your bones. This works best when you start lifting in your teens, but it can happen at any age. Stronger bones means less likelihood of broken bones. That seems like a clear win to me. This win is especially clear when you consider that resistance training is among the safest recreational pursuits you can spend your time on.

The average adult still seems to misunderstand resistance training in younger people. As mentioned in the myth above, you can't avoid resistance. Any kid that runs, jumps, plays outside, walks up and down stairs, or throws a ball will encounter significant and chaotic resistance beyond what you are likely to see in the weight room. Maybe fewer kids are chaotically active these days, but it's still possible that one day they will choose the outdoors over the iPad.

When training in a formal setting, exercises can be progressed under control. They can be used to strengthen muscles, joints and minds without encountering significant risk. Playing virtually any sport will represent more risk to the joints without the same likelihood of controlled progression. This is probably why most people play nothing other than golf and doubles tennis past age 50. The chaos of rec sport is simply too much for unprepared joints. This is an important subpoint: your body can adapt to accommodate just about any insult: preparation is key.

Kids don't necessarily need to set world records with their lifts, but they're already encountering resistance. Kids need to be strong and they need to move well in order to live a better life. Approaching strength gradually and intentionally is exactly what most kids need.

## MYTH: LIFTING WEIGHTS COMPRESSES YOUR SPINE.

So does standing. So does being alive on a planet with gravity. Sitting compresses your spine even more than standing...how much sitting do you do? Poor posture leads to unbalanced spinal compression...how perfect is your posture? Do you intend to hide from gravity by lying in bed the rest of your life? The alternative is to make your body stronger so that it better resists the compressive forces we face all day, every day.

The point of learning to move and lift properly is to learn to master and distribute the forces acting on your body. Control the forces when you can. Prepare yourself for any and all forces in every way you can.

MYTH: RESISTANCE TRAINING IMMEDIATELY MAKES YOU LOOK LIKE A BODYBUILDER. YOU CAN ABSOLUTELY WAKE UP ONE MORNING HAVING BUILT FOREHEAD MUSCLES AND MASSIVE ARMS OVERNIGHT.

This is the tragic story of Arnold Schwarzenegger. That poor guy accidentally lifted a heavy barbell one time. He woke up the next morning as a bulging mass of muscle. Wait, what?

Whether or not you consider bodybuilding a sport, those people work *hard*. They may not always work smart, but damn do they work hard. You don't put on size by accident. If you intend to get bigger, you'd better train specifically for that goal and with significant intensity. Even then, you'll need the genetics to get you there.

You can be strong as hell and still look like a normal human being. If you want to look more like an athletic or curvy human being you can train for that too. However, you won't accidentally stumble into these things. You can have the adaptations you want if you know how to get them. You can avoid the adaptations you don't want if you are training specifically for your goals.

# MYTH: LIFTING MAKES YOU TIGHT, STIFF AND INFLEXIBLE.

This one is pushed by those that don't lift. You know, your yogi, therapist or hipster friend that's never lifted a weight and knows nothing about resistance training? Thankfully this myth is completely untrue. When you lift a weight, muscle fibres contract: shortening, lengthening, and holding position are three different muscle actions we encounter regularly. When you lower the weight, the muscle lengthens. They become strong and proficient at moving through that range of motion. They don't freeze in position just because they got stronger.

If you choose your loads, range of motion and techniques well, lifting will give you mobility you didn't know you had. Countless cases of chronic tension, restriction and pain that I've dealt with in the clinic needed strength above all else. Without adequate strength, your body will freeze you in a cocoon of protective tension that you'll never escape through stretching. Lift well and you'll be able to show off your flexibility anytime, anywhere.

There are even studies out now that have compared resistance training to stretching for building mobility. In these studies, resistance training typically matches or outperforms stretching.

Many of the negative ideas about resistance training are simply unfounded. Much of the time these ideas ideas are based on a lack of understanding, a lack of awareness of the scientific literature, or simply an aversion to hard gym work.

If you encounter these negative ideas, question them. Question them the same way you'd question the positive ideas. If you're unsure whether an idea is true or false, investigate it further rather than accepting the convenient answer.

Much of the negative rhetoric around resistance training comes from gym anecdotes. These gym anecdotes - and videos - feature idiots trying to lift something they shouldn't. There are stupid people in every pursuit. We all have stupid moments. If you keep a level head in the gym, resistance training is incredibly safe.

Now that you're armed with lots of reasons to get over your fear of resistance training, I hope you have an open mind. I hope you can see yourself performing some basic exercises every day and dramatically improving your quality of life. Wait a second, exactly what improvements are we talking about?

We're granted many gifts from resistance training. Some of the most prominent of these gifts are listed here:

Gift: Everything in life becomes a little easier.

I make a point of observing the typical adult performing normal daily movement whenever I can. I'm curious. I want to know what a normal adult needs to do in order to get their shoes on. I want to know how much of a struggle it is for them to pick up a piece of furniture. I want to know because I don't ever need to consider these things in my own life.

The greatest gift you can receive from diligent lifting is a widening and deepening of your scope of capacity. Do you need to rock back and forth to launch yourself out of bed in the morning? Can you easily get down to the ground to play with grandkids, kids or pets? Do you have to be mindful of what you buy in the store because you're unsure about how you'll get it into your house? Do you avoid untying your shoes because you don't know if you'll be able to tie them again? With smart resistance training, you can wipe these concerns off of your radar.

When you're strong through the full range of motion of your joints, the activities of daily living become a breeze. You can bend down anywhere without the support of a wall or step to tie your shoes. You could rearrange your living room with no help. Any movement you were unsure about before can be made accessible.

The movements in your day that you already perform, like climbing stairs, become easier. They may have been challenging at some point. They may have even winded you. They won't anymore.

33

The muscles that propel you through these movements are stronger now, so you only need to use a fraction of their capacity rather than using all of the available muscle fibres. Instead of leaving you exhausted, you'll find yourself with more time to think about more important things. Or daydream. Whatever floats your boat.

It's worth mentioning that the average adult is completely unaware how much of their bandwidth they waste on these concerns. The flash of concern about moving heavy furniture, climbing stairs or bending to put on shoes seems trivial. These concerns add up. They bring about as much cognitive fatigue as they do physical fatigue. Remove the concerns and you'll have CPU available for more important tasks. For example: anything else.

GIFT: YOU CAN LEAVE PAIN BEHIND.

Not all pain. Pain is incredibly complex. However, the aching back and knees can become concerns of the past. The back and the knees are the perfect example because they're almost always the result of poor strength and stability in the core and hips.

What about your herniated disc, though? Surely we can't fix that? No, we can't. We aren't surgeons. However, more than half of adults over age 40 have herniated discs. As high as 20% of teens have herniated discs. Do you hear this many people complaining about them? No...because pain is complex.

One truth about pain is that it functions as an alarm: it's a threat detection system. A tight and weak lower back will ring the alarm bell all day and night, keeping you in pain, to remind you that this important piece of your spine is in danger. The best way to turn off the alarm is to show the nervous system that the danger is no longer present. In this case, that means strengthening the core, hips and lower back so that both mobility and stability are optimal. If you do this, there's no reason for the tissues to feel pain. This is even part of the process to reduce symptoms for a truly severe disc herniation.

Pain is often the body telling you that it has been overused, underused, or otherwise abused and neglected. Give your body a hand. Don't blunt the alarm with rubs, creams and pills without questioning why it's there. Strengthening the body is the best way to show it that there's no need for pain.

35

## GIFT: EVERYTHING IN LIFE BECOMES A LITTLE EASIER.

Have you ever had to do two things in the same day that you really dread? Two things that you knew required your full effort? In these cases, the lesser of the two ends up being okay. It doesn't live up to your expectations of effort or difficulty. This is probably because you have the direct contrast of having something harder to do.

Every day can be like this when you train hard. You don't have to thrash around the gym screaming and foaming at the mouth. Put in an honest, challenging workout early in the day and the rest of the day will seem much easier. Not into working out early? You can still make this principle work for you.

The magic of the workout is partially attributable to endorphins and dynorphins. These brain chemicals that tell you whether you're experiencing euphoria or suffering, respectively. Work out hard and you shut down the dynorphins (the ones that make you feel suffering), and sensitize yourself to endorphins (the ones that make you feel good). What a trade off! Lifting also helps maintain brain-derived neurotrophic factor (BDNF), one of the primary proteins that decreases with aging and cognitive decline. Are you sold yet?

The other mechanism behind this change is your perceived effort. Whatever your workout may be, at some point you will need to pour on the effort in a very clear, direct way. Few things in the rest of your day will require such clear effort. It's not as easy to tolerate a troubled colleague or get through traffic without swearing...we don't know how to best apply our effort. In contrast, the squat is simple and challenging.

When you have a hard workout on your agenda, it puts these other trivial concerns into perspective. Does it really matter what office politics are taking place around you when you can compare that to the effort of hoisting a bar off the ground? I promise that the trivial things in life will reveal themselves as such when you work hard enough.

GIFT: TIME TO PRIORITIZE YOU.

This is a common thread in all of my writing, therapy and fitness advice. Yes, you should care for others and help them whenever you reasonably can. However, if you fail to prioritize your own health and wellbeing, you will be the one that needs help eventually.

I first noticed this trend in the clinic. I often worked on the 'strongest' people in their respective families. These were the people taking care of everyone else and picking up the endless slack wherever it appeared. Strength is a good quality, but it's also finite. You can't express all of your strength 24/7. Many of these people wouldn't take five minutes out of their day to perform an exercise that could erase their pain. Sound familiar?

I would love for you to be selfless, but you need strength to be selfless. You need a lot of strength. You need time to build and recharge that strength. In this case, physical strength helps but is only the beginning.

Make your exercise a ritual. Start that ritual by putting on your headphones, driving to the gym, or hitting a preferred mobility exercise with some clear intentions. Make sure you know: when the ritual begins, it's your time. You may have interruptions. That's okay. The ritual continues whether or not you have to quickly put out a fire. This ritual is all about you. It's about making yourself strong, improving your mindset and your life. Commit yourself to a set amount of ritual time everyday. You'll be better able to help anyone and everyone that needs your strength if you do this.

You can also just pretend that you're a cyborg that doesn't need help, strengthening or a recharge. If you turn out to be less-than-cyborg, you'll just have to build yourself up much more slowly in a clinical setting compared to the gym. It's better to build than rebuild. It's better to get strong before you experience injury or burnout, rather than after.

The choice is yours. Give yourself a hand.

# Gift: Quality of life.

This gift deserves hundreds of sections and chapters to itself. Almost everything about strength training has a positive effect on your quality of life. Unfortunately, we have become longevity focused creatures without the ability to see context. I blame TV doctors peddling magic supplements that allegedly allow you to live to age 400. Age 400 will only cost you $39.99 per month...what a steal!

Cut the crap. Do you want to live to age 400 if 340 of those years are spent in the hospital? Is it worth it to live to 100 if the last 40 years of your life on Earth are spent immobilized and in pain? Apply some context to your fear of death. It's probably natural to fear death, but I think we should be just as motivated by death-in-life.

As you age, your world will shrink a little. This happens early; even as the young professional starts a career. You give up a walk in the park for overtime hours. You give up your rec hockey for a night in front of the TV. You don't even get recess anymore.

Take this trend into middle age and retirement age and it becomes a little more steep. You don't get a dog because you don't know if you can do the necessary walking. You don't travel and see the things on your bucket list because they'll also require walking. You don't stay overnight at a friend's house because your back is acting up. You can't drive anywhere for the same reason. You can't even play simple games with kids and grandkids because you haven't taken care of yourself. Wouldn't it make sense to put off this shrinkage for as long as possible?

Your world will probably shrink and shrivel at some point, unless you are in fact the cyborg mentioned above. How fast it shrinks and when it shrinks is largely up to you. If you're okay with simply plugging your consciousness into your computer and living through facebook and Netflix for the coming decades, so be it. Just keep in mind that as you hide from your lack of capacity you're also hiding from a great and fascinating real world that is dying for some interaction.

We have senses for a reason. I think they're a gift that tells us one thing; we're meant to experience as much as we can. That means good things and bad things. If you have the ability to experience more and you willingly disregard it, it's a tragedy. Staying strong and mobile for as long as possible will keep your quality of life high. Again, cyborgs can ignore this point - cyborgs probably can't feel and experience, anyways - but the rest of us would do well to keep the quality of life in mind as much as quantity.

GIFT: CLOTHES WILL ALWAYS FIT BETTER.

It's a weird phenomenon. Somehow, changing the shape underlying your drapery improves the lay of the drapery. Referring back to the myth above, you'll recall that you won't immediately look like the Incredible Hulk from lifting weights. That's actually impossible, as I'm sure you're aware that the Hulk is a fictional character. If you're thinking the Lou Ferrigno Hulk, that'll also be impossible for most of us, as it takes special genetics and crazy training to stand 6'4 with 23" biceps. I wouldn't worry about that happening to you.

However, if you add a little muscle and subtract a little fat - scale this statement according to your needs - you tend to look better regardless of what you're wearing. If you're a little stronger where it counts, you'll probably stand with a little better posture as well.

People notice these things. If you want to get lost in a crowd, own a mediocre body and stand with crappy posture. You'll blend in like a chameleon. If you meet an old friend for coffee and walk in with solid bearing and an athletic physique, the room might actually start revolving around you.

This isn't entirely about vanity. We have instincts for these things. We can tell when someone is in pain by how they stand and walk, even if you aren't a therapist. We can also tell when someone has put in work on their body, respects themselves and is the epitome of health and vitality. Which would you rather look like?

*The Laws of Strength*

Gifts for the masses! Muscle mass in the right places is a gift. You could write a series of books on the benefits of lifting, so I am going to stop myself there. The point of this chapter is simply to show you that no matter where you are, who you are, or how you feel, lifting can likely improve things for you. Even more importantly, it can improve multiple facets of your life.

Lifting is for everyone. It always has been. Since the dawn of time we've needed to lift things in order to survive. We're faced with a similar reality now. We may not be fleeing predators, but we have couches and electronics that are threatening to turn us into painful bowls of gelatin.

Don't be a bowl of gelatin. Read on. Decide on the body you want and stick with me as I show you how to get it. Even if you've had negative experiences with exercise in the past, there's work you can and should be doing for your own sake.

Daily activity and walking simply don't cut it. Your quality of life is going to be proportional to the work you put in NOW. I'm sorry to those that didn't have the resources to learn about this work sooner, but there's no time like the present. We're all being faced with similar challenges; we all need to do something to address them.

*The Laws of Strength*

# CHAPTER II

# WHO NEEDS TO LIFT?

Are you really still unsure about lifting weights? Aren't you the hesitant one. Or maybe you're lifting weights and don't know if I'm going to show you anything new? Whether you're a seasoned lifting veteran or a frail novice, I've got something for you.

If your mind isn't made up about resistance training yet, read the mock case studies listed below and see if you fit into one of these categories. These scenarios are based on real-world clients, and they'll show you that resistance training really is for everyone.

CASE #1: THE BODYBUILDER/POWERLIFTER/EXPERIENCED LIFTER THAT FEELS FAIRLY CONTENT WITH THEIR TRAINING.

**Subject:** Jake is a 28 year old bodybuilder that is thinking about competing in powerlifting too. His physique is great, but could always be improved. He is also fairly strong in an absolute sense, being able to put up big numbers in the big lifts. Jake's joints creak and crack, his back is usually tight and achy, and he seems to have plateaued on his big lifts.

**Intervention:** Jake needs to learn the most basic forms of periodization and implement them. He feels advanced in the gym compared to the average person so he mindlessly jumps from one professional bodybuilder's program to the next. He also bases his weights and reps around 'feel', as many bodybuilders do.

The 'secret' most bodybuilders would kill for is the way to make continual muscle and strength gains. This isn't actually a secret at all. This is periodization 101, which is the way to apply basic programming principles to training days, weeks and months in order to continually squeeze out more progress.

Despite the long hours many bodybuilders and powerlifters log in the gym, they often overlook this basic concept. The irony is that periodization underpins all long-term resistance training progress. As in many fields, skip the basics and you'll struggle at some point.

47

Jake doesn't need to find a new pursuit. He doesn't need to replace all of his exercises with 'secret' exercises. He doesn't need a 'secret' supplement. He needs to employ basic planning in a way that allows him to understand where his progress comes from.

Jake also has some noisy joints and an achy back. Some people think that this is just part of the iron game. Sometimes it is, and sometimes it isn't. These symptoms could be signs of underlying dysfunction. Jake likely needs to improve both exercise selection and exercise execution top better balance his training stressors. If he implements the basics of stability, mobility, and exercise execution covered later, his achy back and noisy joints will complain a lot less.

CASE #2: THE MIDDLE-AGED WOMAN WITH ZERO LIFTING
EXPERIENCE AND DECLINING PHYSICAL PERFORMANCE.

**Subject:** Barb is a 45 year old woman. She's a mother of two
grown kids. She works a standard work week in a standard office
with a standard desk and a sub-standard computer. Barb has never
done any resistance training in her life, unless you count the aerobics
she saw on TV and the occasional Zumba class. We don't count that.

Barb doesn't feel weak, but she comments on aging a lot. She
often remarks that she can't do as much physical work in the garden
as she used to, or go for long hikes anymore. She used to play tennis
with the family as well, but now she can't play more than 20 minutes
without exhaustion, aches or pain. Barb has tried increasing her daily
step count and taking the stairs at work. Both of these interventions
led to achy knees.

Barb doesn't want to sit back and watch the aging process
happen to her, but everyone tells her that aging is a normal thing.
Barb doesn't want to accept these lifestyle changes, and she hasn't
decided to settle with her circumstances just yet.

**Intervention:** Barb desperately needs to be stronger. Aging
decreases both muscle and bone mass, but this change is
significantly delayed and significantly lessened with resistance
training. These physiological changes typically occur step-for-step
with decreases in physical activity. Above all else, Barb needs to

realize that accepting the strength and performance losses from 'aging' is the worst thing she can do.

Barb is still young. She has plenty of time to get stronger. Barb would be best served by working on some basic bodyweight movements that will increase her strength, coordination and conditioning without throwing her right into heavy lifting. If Barb can increase the strength of her biggest muscle groups, she'll see improvements in endurance, bone density, energy levels and her ability to whoop her kids at tennis.

A common approach to training for middle-aged women is to perform low-intensity cardio or some type of group fitness focused around steps or aerobics movements. None of these will make her significantly stronger. These interventions may actually contribute to accelerated muscle-loss. Barb needs strength, and she needs to find it in a way that doesn't hurt her. Well-performed bodyweight exercises are a great way to safely attain that strength.

CASE #3: THE ELDERLY MAN THAT WORKED HARD PHYSICALLY UNTIL RETIREMENT, BUT HAS BEEN LARGELY INACTIVE SINCE.

**Subject:** Joe is a 71 year old former labourer. He spent his career in the trades, and worked hard physically every day. He never felt the need for the gym, probably due to his generation's perspective on training and the physical nature of his work. Joe was always strong, but his strength has rapidly declined since retiring. He now has trouble golfing and sitting at the card table for more than an hour with friends before his back acts up.

Joe has only been to the doctor a handful of times in his life. He's never been to a physical therapist. He's never set foot in a gym before. He doesn't care much about his physique, but he only begrudgingly accepts the excess weight he's accumulated since retiring. Damn aging.

Joe also has grandkids now. He always wrestled with his kids and taught all of them to play baseball. His grandkids are getting older, and he wants to enjoy sports and playing with them as well. The last time he picked up a baseball off the ground his back went 'out', so he's afraid of doing anything other than watching them play right now.

**Intervention:** Joe needs a daily practice. He doesn't need to set world records or build impressive-looking muscle. He needs real world strength and resilience that carries over to everyday life and rec sports. In 10-20 minutes per day, Joe can dramatically improve his strength, loosen his back, and tolerate playing with the grandkids.

Joe is another candidate for daily bodyweight training. He can make a small investment in his own well being every day, and his physical performance and resilience will increase dramatically. We don't want to treat him like a bodybuilder or a powerlifter. We just need a small piece of each morning to get his strength to levels that support his functional goals.

CASE #4: THE YOUTH ATHLETE WITH COMPETITIVE GOALS.

**Subject:** Ashley is a 14 year old hockey player. Her goal is to play for Team Canada at the Olympics and she's been told that she has the talent. She really wants to improve her game but has already maxed out her ice time. Her parents don't want her lifting weights because they heard this will turn her into a male steroid using bodybuilder with deformed growth plates.

Ashley is young and healthy, but as a competitive athlete she is accumulating imbalances in her body: most team sports require some level of imbalance. The demands of the sport have changed her posture for the worse and she doesn't seem to have the strength to assume good posture. This is starting to affect her on the ice, as her back tightens up and burns with longer skating sessions.

**Intervention:** Ashley *needs* better posture, and postural strength. She's still physically developing, and her body is highly adaptive at this age. The postures and imbalances she experiences now will be more difficult to change later in life.

Ashley is already strong. She's hockey-strong. In terms of daily function she's weak: she isn't strong enough to maintain proper posture, which would reduce the strain on her back. The imbalances of being a competitive athlete are holding her in bad positions. Make no mistake, most sport creates imbalances. Whether these imbalances cause problems or not is less certain.

Ashley needs an off-ice program for a couple of reasons. She wants to improve her performance but has maxed out her sport-skills time. That leaves only indirect physical improvement on the table. She can improve performance, get rid of her aching back and assume good posture with the right combination of exercises. We want to use some regular resistance training to level out her imbalances. This will work as injury-proofing, performance enhancement and it'll improve daily function.

She may play for Team Canada, but she needs to live a good life after that as well. Since Ashley is a rank beginner with resistance training, she needs to start out by training basic capacities and movements. She won't need specialized machines, contraptions or training facilities.

CASE #5: AVERAGE, LOOKING TO BECOME ABOVE-AVERAGE.

**Subject:** Most people aren't super heroes, pro athletes or massive bodybuilders. The majority of these people have good basic function; they can move without pain for the most part, play a little bit, and they can move fast and hard in short spurts when they need to. This person could be any age, and this case is meant to emphasize that normal isn't okay.

I've worked with lots of normal people. I've worked with more of them in the clinic than I do in the gym. Many people think that following the basic life plan, playing it somewhat safe and having a little fun is a good way to go. What most people don't realize is that everyday life with everyday duties is debilitating. Life, gravity and inattentiveness are coming for you.

We like to think that by avoiding lifting and running we keep ourselves safe. The reality is that as life progresses, your capacities regress. The further you get into life moving without conscious thought, without training to remain strong and resilient, the less you'll be able to do over time. As the regression continues, everyday activities become more dangerous. This is the standard non-plan that most people leave school with, and it takes you to the clinic sooner or later.

Life doesn't allow you to play it safe, physically. Even going to the gym and shuffling your way through some token cardio and light resistance training won't cut it. This only provides you with the illusion of covering your bases, when in fact you haven't done enough to stop the regression. Only directed physical work with thoughtful execution can save you from physical decline and eventual pain...sorry!

Modern life is especially punishing on the human body. As mentioned earlier, comfort and technology corrupt us well before our time. Even if you have no competitive or physical aspirations, undoing the damage of everyday life will require some daily effort.

**Intervention:** The best possible outcomes will start with achieving the right mindset. Accept that you don't get a free pass to live everyday life without pain and difficulty. You might get a free ride for a while, but eventually your physical bill will come due. Rather than waiting for it, you can pay the bill in small amounts every day; looking and feeling better all the while.

In this case, you might not desire to be anything greater than a slightly fitter version of yourself, and that's fine. A basic movement practice, performed at least three times per week will give you what you need...though a daily practice is even better. The overall time commitment will need to be the same regardless of how many days you train, so plan on putting in at least one hour per week to start. In ten minutes per day, six days per week, you can accomplish some serious work. This isn't the endgame, but it will get you started.

The examples above should highlight some common problems, as well as some common needs. The human body tends to succeed and fail in similar ways, though we all put our individual spin on the situation. Thanks to our similarities, our common problems have common solutions. This allows us to determine a set of exercise practices that will empower all of us.

Don't worry if I didn't write out your exact situation above. Honestly, there are too many to consider and discuss in a short book. That being said, the solutions to the multitude are actually remarkably similar for several reasons.

For example, back pain is often a glute and core weakness, structural imbalance and stiffness in the low back, hip flexors and hamstrings. These things may cause pain...or they may cause you to move less, to fear movement, and to worry more, which may cause pain.

Knee pain often follows a similar pattern, with some of the stiffness, weakness and pain reaching further down the chain. IT Band symptoms follow the same pattern, as do rounded shoulders with tight traps and neck muscles. Pain in your feet? Better check your hips and core.

The most powerful lesson I learned in the clinic is illustrated above. We may have individual frames and circumstances, but the body tends to fail in remarkably similar ways. When it does, the way we experience pain and dysfunction is largely based on the other factors in our life. The desk worker feels the above patterns as low back pain, while the pro athlete may feel alright up until they tear their

ACL. Similar patterns can be linked to chronic headaches, disc bulges, back pain, sciatica, golf and tennis elbow, and even TMJ (jaw) pain.

In all of these cases, strength becomes an antidote. Strength in the appropriate places alleviates tension, provides stability and mobility, and increases the quality of movement. While stretching may temporarily alleviate pain, it won't fix the problem because it is a weak intervention. Icing, popping pills and saying prayers all operate on the same hope; the hope that something beyond your understanding will fix the problem. It probably won't. To keep the pain away forever, you will need to get stronger.

If you aren't in pain, good for you! This is a good time to build. Whenever you have such a time in your life, you owe it to yourself to prepare for the future. Typically, when we feel good we tend to relax a little. Physical therapy tends to end the same way; you quit when you're feeling good. However, things won't always stay 'good' on their own. Intercept your future problems before they come to the surface.

Lifting is for everyone, and so is strength. Regardless of how strong you currently are, we need to make sure that strength truly makes you bulletproof moving forward. Only then can you chase butterflies, climb mountains and play with your dog, kid, or yoyo. Survival and the ability to thrive exist on the same scale; working towards one will indirectly help the other. Whether you're looking to get out of pain or looking to set world records, read on.

*The Laws of Strength*

*The Laws of Strength*

# THE LAWS OF STRENGTH

No more messing around. Everything you've read to this point will give you some context on what you're about to read. The Laws are to be followed by everyone interested in getting stronger. Some are more important than others, but all are important. Honour the laws and you honour your body and mind.

Understand that the laws are principles: they apply across different circumstances. Whether you're a competitive powerlifter or a lifelong couch potato, the laws operate in a field of relativity. Apply them to your own context and circumstances, regardless of the magnitude of goal, exercise or load being lifted.

Methods come and go. The specific methods you use all need to operate on sound principles. The Laws are the principles that underscore any good program, pursuit or method in fitness.

*The Laws of Strength*

# Law #1: Know Thyself

The ancient Greek axiom has seen many uses, all of which suited the current user. In our case, we can use this wisdom in several meaningful ways. The axiom is important in the development of both the body and the mind. It's most useful when you remember that development of the body and mind go hand in hand.

Knowing yourself requires different levels of focus.

First, you must know what your current strengths and weaknesses are. Make a physical list - put pen to paper, or fingers to keyboards - to delineate these strengths and weaknesses. Before you ever perform a movement evaluation or test, you should be aware of what you struggle with and what assets you have. You're bombarded with this data all day, every day. All you have to do is pay attention.

In your list, make sure you include everything you want to change. In this case, excess bodyweight can be a weakness. Categorizing the weight in such a way makes it a little easier to confront on a daily basis.      Weaknesses can be diverse, such as pain or the inability to perform a certain movement or activity. Picking up kids, squatting, running,carrying groceries, the conditioning required for a hiking vacation are all good examples.

If you can't do it comfortably yet you need to do it, it's a weakness. If your legs shake every time you climb the steps into the gym, we can safely assume core, hip, or leg strength is a weakness.

If you're a powerlifter, athlete or experienced lifter, write down what you know you need to improve. If your deadlift lags behind your squat, label it a weakness. If you sprain your ankle five times per season, ankle strength, stability and mobility are likely a weakness. Be as specific as possible.

Conversely, strengths can be physical or otherwise. If you know you have weight to lose, your frustration and determination can become a strength. The biggest changes and improvements come from uncomfortable situations. Find your strengths wherever you can; the squat, bench press, specific body parts, willpower, your schedule, your family support, etc.

These strengths and weaknesses represent your capacity. They tell you what you can and can't do in the present moment. These are the boundaries you will need to push. An increase in general capacity means a functional carryover to sport and everyday life. An increase in the specific capacity you need right now can change your life.

If you know these things starting out, you know what you need to improve. You know what you need to monitor as you work. You know what strengths you can use to attack your weaknesses. Before you do anything, you need to know what you're currently capable of.

Knowing yourself also means knowing *how* you move. Pay attention the next time you hit a workout, the next time you climb the stairs, the next time you sit in a chair for any length of time. Do you fall into any bad habits? Does one knee or leg behave differently than the other when doing these things? This data is crucial to your longevity as a functioning and physical person.

The squat is an excellent movement to use for discovering bad habits. When performing the squat, we immediately see if you put weight on each leg equally, if one hip is tight, if one ankle is restricted, if the lower back or core is weak, and if your overall mobility is good or problematic. We can determine this all from one movement.

It's your responsibility to investigate these things on your own. Therapists and coaches can't follow you around all day, every day, correcting every posture and movement. Ultimately, you need to know your body better than anyone else. Get a professional assessment and watch the videos in later sections to help determine what your strengths and weaknesses may be.

Look at your circumstances objectively. Leave your ego and your opinion out of it. Can you squat deep without pain or movement compromise? Can you perform all of your current exercises with relative symmetry? Analyze where you are, and keep that position in mind as you move forward. Without knowing your own body, it's habits, movements, strengths and weaknesses, any physical intervention is doomed to fail. Know Thyself. All of Thyself. Then change thyself if thou needs to.

## ACTION

Test your abilities. Be present as you move throughout your day, and through your workout. Do you encounter tights spots? Do you have pain? Which movements do you find most challenging? You don't need to be an anatomist or an exercise physiologist. You do need to be an expert on your own body.

Record these findings in an exercise log from day to day, and be as objective as possible. Record your movement quantities: the sets, reps, durations and weight on the bar. Record your movement qualities: how deep you squat, or how the range of motion, the presence or absence of pain, your subjective stability, and so forth.

Feel isn't objective, but subjective changes often occur before the ones we can measure objectively. Squats will typically feel better before they get deeper. The more information you record, the clearer your direction will become.

*The Laws of Strength*

## LAW #2: PATIENCE

Patience is the least appreciated virtue. Like flossing and eating vegetables, it's something everyone in the world recommends but very few people act on. One way or another, life will instruct you on the value of patience. You can choose to observe that value as it pushes you toward your goals, or you can observe it in hindsight as something you should've done.

In physical training, patience is the only way forward. The *only* way. Impatience in the gym or in any fitness pursuit will lead you to plateaus and pain. This isn't coincidence, it's physiology. The body responds and adapts to stimuli that don't destroy it. Lifting a weight that's heavy but manageable will allow you to adapt and grow stronger. Lift a weight that's too heavy for your current capacities and something will pop. This is essentially how all exercise-related injuries occur. If you're pushing your boundaries, you might survive and grow stronger. If you ignore your boundaries and you're unprepared for the task at hand, you could get hurt.

This might tempt you to play it safe and never engage in any exercise. Remember that although avoidance seems safer, it means that you're patiently waiting for time to hurt you rather than experimenting on your own. Time will hurt all of us, but it will hurt the weak ones first. Don't be one of the weak ones. Though skipping the gym may seem safer, it only delays the inevitable. You need to confront your weaknesses to prevent them from running your life.

Modern life revolves around speed. Technology has provided us the luxury of instant access, instant online shopping, and instant gratification. From fast food to Netflix, we have the world at our fingertips at any given time. Information is always passing in front of our eyes, and answers are never out of arm's reach thanks to our incredible google-machines.

Even weight loss books aren't sold with promises of sustained success; instead they promise you can lose a substantial amount of weight in three weeks. They know you hate delayed gratification and waiting for results.. Fitness books are the same, promising superhuman results overnight.

All of our luxuries have reduced our capacity for waiting. I don't think the human hardware has changed, only the software that operates it. We have the ability to express patience, and we should.

In your own physical practice, this means committing to mastering movements. This is no small task, and it will keep you busy. Committing yourself to mastery will allow you to make continual progress right up to your genetic potential. If instead you take a shortcut, you've doomed yourself to encounter an immovable obstacle in the near future.

For example, if you stick with the basic bodyweight squat until your good enough to do it while sleeping upside down and blindfolded, you'll be a great squatter. While learning to do that you probably made physical progress, both in strength and physique. Now that you've mastered the squat, all you need to do is find ways to exceed the load your body is accustomed to. If you can keep your technique consistent, you can increase load safely for a long, long time.

If your clone decided to rush through their squat practice, they would've gotten to weighted squats faster than you. They probably gave into their existing imbalances because they didn't care to master their technique. With existing imbalances hurting their technique they'll undoubtedly see those imbalances WORSEN. Even worse, they'll never get the same physique or strength results as you in the long run. Eventually, their only option will be to return to step one and master the technique. Sadly, the ego will likely prevent this from happening for most people; it seems like too much of a step back.

While patience may seem overrated on the surface, you can see that a little patience now will save you lots of trouble down the road. Challenge yourself to overcome your technique problems and make steady progress, rather than transforming overnight. You can still progress quickly, just make sure you're earning your progression rather than rushing it.

A lack of patience and understanding is among the primary reasons experienced lifters get stuck. They don't care enough to journal or log their workouts, record their weights and make small changes. If they did, they wouldn't need secret exercises, programs and supplements.

Patience is a basic skill that must be mastered. Play the long game. Have a long term plan. Make small, incremental improvements in your technique, exercise selection and weights used. Small changes. Incremental changes. Step by step improvement. This is how big goals are attained.

Patience in your physical practice is not only necessary for your long term success and health, it's also rewarding. We're often so busy rushing to accomplish things that we forget to enjoy the journey. Believe it or not, it's enjoyable to learn about your own body, feel out your movements and exercises, and experiment with your technique. It's also fun to perform something slightly more challenging than you did the week before; this way you're always making some progress. This is the heart and soul of periodization, which we'll cover a little later.

## ACTION

Record everything. Write down what you do each training session and note how it feels. Do this for at least two weeks consistently. By recording your work inputs, you'll know what you need to do to make progress on a weekly basis. At the end of each training week, look over your training log and reflect on the progress you made.

Progress is rarely sweeping, dramatic, or outstanding...especially on a small timescale. Sometimes progress is an exercise feeling easier for the same number of sets and reps. Sometimes progress means you accomplished the same workout in less time. Celebrate the small, incremental progress that will lead you to your big goals. Above all else, learn to be happy with 'better', instead of needing to be the best right now.

For bonus points, look for the long term trends in the short time scale. Understand the vision behind your training, and estimate where your current training will take you. After planning appropriately, make sure you accept and enjoy where you are right now. Even if you've got a long way to go, you are where you are. You can only progress as fast as you can progress. Do what you have to do and check all of the necessary boxes.

*The Laws of Strength*

*The Laws of Strength*

*The Laws of Strength*

# LAW #3: AGGRESSION

You've arrived at law number three. Depending on your training experience and personality type, you're either thinking, "Yeah, bro!", or, "Wait, what?". Don't jump to any conclusions just yet: keep in mind that this law only works if you adhere to all of the other laws as well.

The theory behind resistance training is nice. The idea of adapting to a controlled stress doesn't seem all that bad. Heck, lifting weights doesn't seem like it'll be much work if you train within your limits and utilize Patience (Law #2).

The harsh reality of progression is that you're always pushing your body to adapt. It wants to survive, and in many ways the body operates as though you're still a nomad sleeping on the plains and eating three berries per day. In this environment, getting stronger isn't much of a reality and it isn't a positive adaptation. When starvation is a legitimate threat, the body doesn't want you seeking extra work to gain extra muscle. This would be the definition of inefficiency, and in our distant past it would have been a bad thing.

You aren't much of a nomad anymore. Your incidental activity levels are much lower, and your food and sustenance sources are abundant. You even have memory foam slippers. Your survival isn't immediately at risk, even if your body acts as though it is. It's this throwback quality that makes gaining muscle and strength a challenge.

The patient application of resistance will take you a long way, but that resistance needs to challenge your body if you want to adapt. Your workouts need to be challenges to the system, challenges that can be perceived as threats. For most people, sets of 80 reps with pink dumbbells won't cut it.

You need to express some controlled aggression, within your capacity. Aggression doesn't mean foaming at the mouth, screaming and listening to death metal. In fact, any '**overly assertive behaviour in the pursuit of one's goals**' could be considered aggressive. If you aren't being overly assertive, your body won't pay any attention. If you put yourself through a workout and your body didn't notice, it has no incentive to adapt in any direction. Too many people spin their tires at the gym, not accomplishing any real work with their time. Without results, the gym becomes less appealing.

You need to know your capacity and your boundaries. In knowing these things, you need to subtly push them with your work. You need to be assertive in working towards goals, mastering movements, and pushing your resistance. Otherwise, the body will not change. Remember: if the body isn't disturbed a little, nothing will happen.

Most people have lingering aggression that needs to be 'worked out' anyways. While it'd be nice to float the bullshit of everyday life and the struggles of dealing with people and work, that may not be realistic for you. Many people turn into masochistic savages when you hand them a dumbbell, even when seconds earlier they were talking about a baby shower they just attended.

Being aggressive in the gym or during a workout doesn't mean trying to set records every time you break a sweat. It doesn't mean shaking and screaming to hit your reps. It means knowing what's necessary for adaptation, and knowing what you're capable of. Above all else, it means employing tenacity to push your boundaries, rather than hiding from them on the couch.

Your everyday life can teach you to hold back. Socially it's better to err on the side of being polite or generous than it is to be aggressive. Being aggressive at work might earn you an indefinite, unpaid period of time off (otherwise known as unemployment). This doesn't mean aggression is bad, it simply means that it requires the right application.

Assertive behaviour can also be applied to things that we think of as passive. You can attack your rest and recovery goals as much as your exercise goals. Rest and recovery are crucial for physical progress, but most of us work hard in the gym then phone-in the whole rest and recovery part. Aggressively pursuing better sleep hygiene - sleep routines, regular bedtime, dark room, etc - will be just as important for hitting long term goals as what you do in the gym. Mastering your breathing and your ability to relax between exercises and workouts is just as crucial. You need to aggressively pursue development in all areas.

## ACTION

Find your aggressive side. Attach a switch to that side, and learn to turn it on and off. When it's time to make progress at something, it's time for some controlled and intelligent aggression. Getting stronger means making progress, so you'll need to attack your practice with some conviction. Accept that progress requires effort. Intelligent effort applied close to your current limits is exactly the target to shoot for.

Without applying any aggression, we never move the needle. We can spend days, weeks, or years spinning our tires. We need to commit to our goals, and commit to the work required. Aggressively pursue improvement in any way you can, and don't be shy about it.

*The Laws of Strength*

# LAW #4: PROGRESSION

Since the dawn of human storytelling, we've had access to tragic stories. A good tragedy awakens uncomfortable emotions that can leave you pondering dark thoughts for hours, days or weeks. I hope you can embrace these uncomfortable feelings in your own story when you encounter a lack of progress in training. Rather than hiding from the disappointment of failures, you need to learn to accept that disappointment and resolve to change something.

Surely I'm being dramatic? Whenever I train in a public gym, I observe the utter absence of basic progression principles in the training of both the average person and most trainers. This Law could fill a book on it's own, and it may be more important for long term success than any other exercise principle. I'd be disappointed for you if you spent countless hours without seeing any improvement, but my disappointment wouldn't get you anywhere.

Progression requires you to employ basic strategy to your training. It means that between point A and point B - which could be any timeframe from a one week period to a four year period - you've decided to make a certain amount of progress. Of course said goal and direction must be realistic and objective. The measures that will take you from point A to point B must be considered, and they must be intelligent. If you choose inappropriate measures to get you from A to B, B becomes a dream, not a goal.

As vague as the above sounds, we don't need to add unnecessary complexity to this principle. If the goal is to squat your bodyweight, twice your bodyweight, or thrice your bodyweight - that's right, I used the word thrice - the measures will be similar. You'll need to manage and improve your squat technique. You'll need to manage how much poundage you squat each week. Most importantly, you must ensure that what you do in training can reasonably lead you toward your goal.

While these concepts sound basic, they're routinely ignored by both newbies and 'experienced' lifters alike. For example, many group fitness trainees want stronger legs and a stronger core to help them live a more exciting and capable life outside of the gym. They attend their fitness classes, where the focus is squeezing in more reps in less time, and many won't perform a single proper squat repetition.

Even though they do several hundred 'squats', they haven't practiced an efficient form of the movement one single time. They've just spent an hour screwing with their mechanics, reinforcing imbalances and downgrading their own mobility. Does that sound like an intervention that will lead to any worthwhile point B?

You can also look at an 'experienced' lifter. People often get offended when I call them novices in our training sessions, but I'm left with no choice. These novices may win competitions, hit some of their goals, and have an attractive physique....but they have no clue how they did it other than putting in hard work. They haven't employed the most basic rules of progression. If you haven't outgrown the novice methods for hitting goals, you're still a novice.

You may be wondering why you'd bother with this Law if you can have some success without it. That seems a reasonable thought. It'll seem reasonable for about six months to one year. At that point you'll realize you've plateaued and you have no idea how to move forward. At this point it's safe to assume that you've also sacrificed exercise technique to achieve some much needed progress. Your poor joints!

Whether you are a champion or a chump, you *must* implement this Law. Without invoking the Law of Progression, you have no hope of making continual progress. You have no hope of maintaining your progress over time. You're like a leaf blowing aimlessly in the wind. Be the wind, not the leaf. Direct your progress and go wherever you please.

The basic consideration for the Law of Progression is thus:

## Technique must remain a constant, regardless of load.

Your first major project is always to improve your technique as much as possible on an exercise. You'll make tremendous progress just by improving your technique. Hone your optimal technique - aim for perfect, but accept that it doesn't exist in the same way for everyone - and practice that technique often. Think of your workout sessions as chances to practice technique, not to 'work out'...whatever the hell that means. If you add load and your technique changes negatively, you added too much load. Master the technique at your working weight and progress from there.

Remember, ideal technique is ideal because it will give you the most return on investment. Ideal technique means minimizing or controlling joint stress, maximizing muscular stress, and adopting the form that allows you to move the most load. All of these things move you closer to your goals, whatever they may be.

Some exercises require you to 'cheat'. This is okay as long as the technique doesn't destroy your body in the process. Arching in the bench press is a good example of this, as it actually makes the lift safer. This technique seems like a shortcut, but really it's just the best way to perform the lift safely while challenging yourself. Therefore, this is good technique.

Conversely, if you're trying to keep your back flat when you bench press, you probably won't be able to lift as much and you'll get creaky joints much faster. Additionally, if you start with a flat back and arch halfway through a lift because the weight is too heavy, you're just a cheater.

In competitions, form may vary because maximal loads are being tested. That doesn't mean you should train with chaotic form, or that you should push your training weights to this extent routinely. It's better to train with slightly less weight and better form than it is to load up the bar and butcher your technique to get a meager PR.

To ensure your technique is optimal, check out my youtube videos on the primary exercises. Learning good form and learning to practice are invaluable to your success, whatever your goal may be.

# You must do more than you did in your last unit of training time.

This doesn't mean every session requires load progress, though this can happen for beginners. As you get stronger and more experienced, you'll need to look at bigger units of training time. Your goal should be to at least marginally increase one of your training measures - intensity, duration, overall volume, etc - from one block of time to the next.

How does this look for different training goals?

## ENDURANCE TRAINING

Those looking for better lower body endurance can increase the total number of squats they can perform in a session. Week to week this can be advanced. You can increase the length of the session for a few weeks, then decrease it and try to fit the same reps into less time.

86

This means an increase in the density of your session: you can perform more work per unit of time. When training for endurance, usually the goal is to achieve more in less time, or to be able to sustain efforts for longer blocks of time.

You could also simply expand the overall volume of a session, as one would do with walking, running or total reps of squats. This demonstrates a systemic increase in endurance capacity at the same intensity.

When discussing endurance in the world of resistance training, the measurement is typically your number of reps performed. Performing the same exercise, with the same load, for more reps means an increase in endurance. Decreasing the amount of time it takes you to perform this number of repetitions represents an increase in your speed-endurance.

Whatever your preferred measurement, you need to push to increase your workload. Whether that's an increase in your speed-endurance or your systemic endurance will depend on your goal. Make sure you have a concrete, objective way to track the amount of work you're doing.

## Strength Training

To lift more, you must lift more. From week to week you must find a way to increase the load you overcome. Without increasing load, your body has no reason to adapt and become stronger. You may need to reduce the overall number of reps you perform to increase the weight or difficulty of the exercise. You will likely need to change your reps from week to week, allowing the rep volume (sets multiplied by reps) to ebb and flow between higher and lower reps to achieve your gains long term.

Try basic **Linear Progression**. This means that for each primary exercise in each week of training, you attempt to gradually increase the load. That means that on Day 1 of Week 1 you may lift 50lbs, and on Day 1 of Week 2 you will try to do the same sets and reps with 55lbs. Do this until you can't keep up with the added load. When you can't keep up, reduce the load by 10% for the same sets and reps and start the progression cycle again. When this doesn't work, move onto **Double Progression**.

**Double Progression** allows you to manipulate the reps you perform with your working weight on the fly. When simply adding more resistance to an exercise isn't an option - Linear Progression doesn't work forever, unfortunately - you need to find another way to vary the stimulus.

Suppose your linear progression leads you to a plateau in which you can deadlift 100lbs for 3 sets of 5. If you try 105lbs, you can't hit any sets of 5. You've tried backing the weight off and reapproaching, but it hasn't helped you conquer 105. Is that it? Have you reached your potential? Not by a long shot.

*The Laws of Strength*

The most logical change would be to implement basic Double Progression. Instead of always trying for 3 sets of 5 reps, now you'll give yourself a range of repetitions to hit. Now your goal will be to hit 3 sets of **4-6** reps, instead of 5. While this might seem a more broad way of targeting 5 reps, it works differently in practice.

Since you've already mastered 100lbs for 3x5, let's start there. Load up the bar to 100lbs. Now your goal is to get as many reps as you can within the range you've chosen. In this case, we know you can do 3x5 so you'll be trying to get 6 reps in each set instead.

Before your workouts would have looked like this:

- Set 1 = 100 lbs x 5 reps
- Set 2 = 100 lbs x 5 reps
- Set 3 = 100 lbs x 5 reps

But now you have a range to shoot for, not a single number. Now, your goal is to get as many reps in that range as possible. Your first workout would probably look like this:

- Set 1 = 100 lbs x **6 reps**
- Set 2 = 100 lbs x **5 reps**
- Set 3 = 100 lbs x **4 reps**

Given the above example, you've technically only hit the same number of reps as you were getting before. However, the rep range allows you to push harder on each set. Whereas before you may have had energy in the tank after 5 reps, you're now asked to provide your maximal effort on each set, even if that means the reps drop from set to set.

In the next couple of workouts, you'll eek out some new progress. This progress will probably look like this:

- Set 1 = 100 lbs x **6**
- Set 2 = 100 lbs x **5**
- Set 3 = 100 lbs x **5**

Though you may not feel too accomplished with this progress, you should. You only added one rep, but that extra rep just added 100lbs to your total tonnage for the day. This is enough to drive the body toward further adaptation.

When you're able to hit the top number in your rep range for all of your sets, you're ready to add weight to the bar. This is the sneaky benefit of Double Progression. Your last workout at 100lbs will look like this:

- Set 1 = 100 lbs x **6**
- Set 2 = 100 lbs x **6**
- Set 3 = 100 lbs x **6**

That's right, you've maxed out your set and rep targets at 100lbs. This means the 'double' part of Double Progression kicks in:

you add weight to the bar. Your next deadlift workout after the one described above will look like this:

- Set 1 = **105 lbs** x 5
- Set 2 = **105 lbs** x 4
- Set 3 = **105 lbs** x 4

Now you're using the weight you couldn't handle before; this is what resistance training is all about! Your number of sets remains the same, but your reps will reflect the increase in weight; you may only get 4-5 reps per set at 105 lbs. You may get 4's across the board, and that's okay.

Your goal is still to hit 6 reps per set before you increase weight again. Over the coming weeks, you will probably stagger your sets up toward that goal, hitting some sets of 6, some 5's, and some 4's. Provide a solid effort on all of the sets and your body will realize that it needs to get stronger.

Eventually your body will refuse further weight increases again. This is expected, normal, and okay. If we could simply progress in a linear fashion all the time we wouldn't need strength coaches. Rather than attacking the bar in a futile effort to move more weight, it's best to respect when you've met your match and hit the reset button.

If you can't hit the new weight for the rep range you're working with, your body isn't ready for it. You can check your form, but it's likely your body needs extra recovery of its strength producing systems before you can progress further. Pushing the body to adapt is a draining process, leaving you unrecovered from your workouts. While you can sustain progress for a while, eventually the only thing that will help is allowing the system to recover fully.

Perform a 'load reset' by taking 10% of the weight off the bar. It doesn't need to be exactly 10%, just get to the closest possible interval. Perform the same number of sets with the same repetition range as you previously worked with. With a bar that's 10% lighter, the top repetition number in the rep range should come easily to you, or at least easier than the weight you were attempting. This decrease in load does a few important things:

- It allows you to reinforce proper form with an easier weight.
- It allows your body to recover from previous workouts, as the weight isn't as challenging.
- It keeps you lifting, making sure that you're maintaining your progress while recovering.
- It automatically increases your lifting volume again, allowing you to spark some new growth. Before you'd been stalled out at sets of 4's, now you'll be able to hit sets of 6 again with ease thanks to the lighter                                      weight.

The math, for those interested, looks like this:
- Before the stall volume = 2 sets of 4, 1 set of 3 @ 105 lbs = 11 total reps multiplied by 105 lbs. **Tonnage/session = 1155 lbs**

■ After the reset volume = 3 sets of 6 @ 95 lbs (105 lbs minus 10%) = 18 total reps multiplied by 95 lbs. **Tonnage/session = 1710 lbs**

By the time you return to the weight you'd stalled at before, you'll have had plenty of recovery time and lots of good reps in the tank. This time, you'll be able to hit the bottom of the rep range for all of your sets. The progression cycle then continues on as it did before.

In the case that you still can't hit that goal weight, you're approaching the end of your time with the current template. You may need to switch up exercises, or simply change up the sets and reps. The best way to do this is to simply increase your goal rep range to include 1-2 fewer reps than you could before. So if your goal range had been 4-6, it will now be 3-6 reps per set. You'll be strong enough to get back into the target range with this change, and your progress will continue as before.

When trying to get stronger, lower rep training is superior to high rep training. This isn't necessarily true for building muscle or increasing endurance, but this is the best way to increase strength in most cases. If your goal is more related to hypertrophy or endurance, you could increase the rep range by 1-2 reps on the top end instead. This would mean changing your target from 4-6 reps to 4-8 reps. This small change can allow you to rack up the extra poundage you need to keep the progress (#gainz) coming.

**Progressing Exercises** is another great way to build progression into your training. Not everyone needs to sling heavy barbells. Some people will prefer to use calisthenics to build their ideal body. This is an excellent route to choose for most people. Even those that would prefer to sling barbells would look and feel better with a little bodyweight training in their routine.

Calisthenics, or bodyweight training, is a combination of several popular disciplines that has many unique methods. This training incorporates movements from yoga, gymnastics training and competition, and essentially any other pursuit that makes intelligent use of body weight as a load.

With a little experience, you'll soon realize that there are many different levels of difficulty built into the exercises themselves. A Pushup is easier than a One-Arm Pushup, but they both use similar muscle groups in similar ways. Between these two pushup variations are dozens of alternative movements that can be used to bridge the gap between the two. Each variation can challenge you in a slightly different way, with slightly more difficulty. By the time you reach the One-Arm Pushup in your progression series, you should be able to tackle that impressive challenge thanks to your progressive approach.

Whether or not you dream of One-Arm Pushups, progressing your efforts through exercise selection is a smart way to train. Utilizing the resistance of the body, you can learn to manipulate leverage to achieve the effect you want. These workouts travel with you anywhere and everywhere. These workouts won't cost you a dime, nor will they require a commute or time to set up equipment. This is the ultimate flexible training system.

This progression will work in both the **simple** and **double** formats. Start with the easiest variations and perform them for the prescribed sets and reps. Always start with the easiest, even if you're already in shape. This allows the muscles, connective tissues and joints to adjust to the new stressors over time.

When the sets and reps are easy for that exercise, move to the next exercise in the progression. Repeat the progression for that exercise until the sets and reps become easy again. When you inevitably stall out at some point, move to **double progression**, giving yourself a repetition range to hit instead.

Bodyweight exercise can build serious muscle if used well. It can also give you a great endurance workout, simultaneous mobility and stability training, and it may build the body in a more balanced way than more reductionist approaches like bodybuilding.

The inter-muscular coordination required - the body functioning as a unit - is a much more sustainable way to train than traditional machine-based resistance exercise. Best of all, calisthenic training is fun. It's cool. If you can picture yourself working up to Single Leg Squats and Single Arm Pushups over time without getting excited, I'd check for a pulse.

Look out for my upcoming project; The Conquest Book of Physical Methods. It will contain detailed steps to follow in the progression of both bodyweight and weighted exercises. Until then, check out my Youtube channel to see the most commonly prescribed exercise progressions in action!

Progressing your exercise selection can happen with traditional gym-exercises as well, but in this case it's closer to a rotation than a progression. For example, a powerlifter may focus on high-bar squats for a while to help boost their low-bar competition squat. Practicing your competition movements is key, but the body does need some variety as well.

Okay, calm down. We can finally talk about building muscle. If you're a bodybuilder, start with implementing the above detailed work for strength and endurance training before getting ahead of yourself. Most people that sign up for training need to simplify, not introduce greater complexity into their training.

Whether you're a bodybuilder or not, I strongly advise you to choose other training and fitness goals as well. Training for size is great if that's your passion, but it shouldn't happen at your physical expense. Choose some mobility, endurance and strength goals to hit along the way to the stage and you'll be glad you did.

For the non-bodybuilder readers, you probably won't need to do much more than what was described in the above sections. Strength training inherently takes care of some growth stimulus, but you're unlikely to turn into Arnold overnight following those methods. This is the perfect compromise for most people.

If building lots of muscle is your primary goal, you'll need some extra firepower in your arsenal. Strength training does cover many of your bases, but you need to know what those bases are to give yourself the best chances of splitting your sleeves.

There are only a few primary factors that lead to Hypertrophy:

**1.    Metabolic Fatigue.** This effect is achieved when the work being performed by the muscle outpaces its ability to supply energy and remove waste products. Every rep, every sprint, every hard sneeze requires significant muscular output. Repeating muscular efforts in quick succession with a challenging load will require massive energy output from your poor muscle cells.

At some point, byproducts of energy production accumulate faster than you can clear them, resulting in acidic hydrogen ions temporarily weakening you and making the muscles burn...this is what most people inaccurately call the lactic acid burn. This energy crisis forces the muscles to adapt to store more energy and grow to provide                         better                         burn-resistance.

Achieve this effect in your workouts by performing higher reps - higher than 10 per set - focusing on fatiguing the muscle as much as possible. Don't worry too much about your inter-set rest, as resting longer - around two minutes - allows you to perform harder sets than resting            less            time            between            sets.


**2.    Muscular Tension.** Contracting a muscle requires maximal tension in the recruited muscle fibres. Overloading the muscles by exposing them to more tension per set and more overall tension per workout - more tonnage lifted, reps performed, weight used - will force them to adapt. Tension stress is a threat to the fibre; tension can rip things. The muscle will adapt by growing stronger and larger to protect itself from that load in the future. This is also why you need to continually push your boundaries; eventually the old loads just won't be threatening enough to create change.

**3.  Muscular Damage.** Your body is like a car that repairs itself with either new and improved parts or scrap from the junkyard. Exercise gives you that 'new and improved' effect. In order to initiate productive repairs, you need to create some extra damage. Your tissues completely recompose themselves in the natural life cycle; cells die and are replaced, eventually replacing entire tissues and organs.

You can drive that repair to specific parts of the body and you can choose the replacement parts by damaging your muscles with tension. As your body lifts a weight, you're creating microtears in the tissues. When the body repairs these tissues, it'll repair them stronger and thicker to avoid future damage. Little does your body know that there are always heavier dumbbells and harder exercise progressions. It would seem that eccentric muscle actions - slow or powerful muscle-lengthening, as in lowering a bar on a biceps curl - create the most damage.

These factors probably describe much of your understanding of training to this point. Most trainees know that incurring some damage, burning muscles, and heavy loads will help them get bigger and stronger. Rather than mindlessly hoping to achieve those effects, use these factors specifically in your workouts to achieve the burn, the loading, or the damage you need to adapt.

Progression is essential to growth. Growth is essential for continuing your functional life. Regardless of your training goals, focus on progression to ensure continual results. You can improve your body composition, strength, and mobility by starting a new routine, or you can incorporate these things into your existing routine by simply tracking your progress and planning for it to continue indefinitely.

## Action

Use an app, an old notebook or your diary to start tracking your physical development. During your workouts, record what you do, how much you do, and how it feels. You don't need to be exact with any of this, but you need a measuring stick to beat in subsequent weeks.

Use whatever format makes the most sense to you; it's your workout log after all. Reflect on your day before bed. If you haven't performed any directed exercise that day, write down the date and the word 'nothing' beside it. Every day is a chance to move forward or fall back. You don't need to run a marathon every day; you just need to make sure that you're controlling your direction.

Bonus points if you take care to record the factors required to make progress. Track your total tonnage or volume from session to session and week to week. Know what you have to do in each training session to spur further adaptation.

*The Laws of Strength*

# LAW #5: REGRESSION

This is the last 'ession' Law, I swear. The last two Laws described ways to march forward and methods to continue that march when progress slows. It'd be nice to march straight forward into continual improvement for the rest of your life, but this isn't realistic.

Walk in a straight line long enough and you'll eventually run into a wall. Or maybe step off a cliff...it depends on the journey you've undertaken. The straight line strategy probably isn't the only one you'll need for continual progress, as the pain of the wall or cliff may suggest.

When walking your straight line and enjoying the rewards you've been reaping, you'll encounter the cliff at some point. Most people ignore it, or simply hope the same strategy will keep working to traverse the coming peaks and valleys. Tsk, Tsk. Rather than stepping into an obstacle you're unprepared for, what if you could stop and consider the obstacle for a moment? What if you could take a step back, adjust your direction, and continue the onward march safely for another length of time? This is the art of regression, and it is necessary for human beings that want continual improvement.

Regression can be forced upon you, or you can decide to use it strategically. If you pretend that you can continually adapt to everything that comes your way, you'll be woefully unprepared for something along your path. Spend enough time in the gym and you'll see this example play out dozens of times. The regulars that once squatted lots of weight now use baby weights. Then they stop squatting and instead use the leg press. Then they can no longer leg press so they sit on the bike for an hour watching sports highlights.

If your gym-mate had the foresight to take one step back, this dramatic regression wouldn't have happened. Recall from the Law of Progression that when we start to stall, we strategically reduce the load being used and repeat our building process at a slower pace. This break from maximal efforts gives us time to recover, reevaluate and perfect technique. The reset allows us to phone-in a few workouts while we find our motivation again. This is a controlled regression. Just like a controlled forest fire, it isn't ideal when compared to unlimited and endless progression, but it is what we need to do.

Your gym-mate is stuck on the bike because he failed to honour his body with some controlled regression. Inevitably the weights will get heavy for you, which is the point of lifting. The absolute weight - the weight on the bar - matters less than your relative effort or closeness to your true max. When the weight gets heavy enough, the challenge of the exercise will exceed your current abilities slightly, forcing your body to compensate. This compensation allows you to survive the set, but it isn't the most efficient or sustainable technique: it's a survival tactic. If you fail to notice this change in technique, the new and uglier squat will become your normal squat.

Compensation patterns exist to allow us to survive our current predicament. After the predicament, we're meant to go back to our

104

normal patterns. In the gym, the compensation can get you a few extra pounds at the expense of your tissues, joints and movement quality. You can probably survive a few sets of this, but eventually it'll wreck you.

It would be much better to keep your form constant and handle less weight. If you can't progress the weight with your current technique, back off and re-approach as discussed earlier. The alternative is adopting a technique that works today and hurts you tomorrow. This is why many people will tell you lifting, deadlifts and squats are dangerous; they didn't pump the breaks and they suck at the movement as a result.

Sometimes your regression will need to be more dramatic. For example, you may need to use some supplementary exercises that don't seem to fit with your new, superhuman body. Before you could squat heavy, you needed the ability to squat your bodyweight with some skill. If at some point in your training you notice you can't squat your bodyweight perfectly anymore, you need to address that. Sure, it seems easy and embarrassing to work on given your progress, but this is a big red flag. Something is off. You may need to address mobility deficits, stability in single leg exercises, or you may need to switch up your primary exercises for a while.

The intervention changes depending on the circumstances. The most important problem-solving steps in this equation are the following:

1.    Pay attention. Step back on your terms or you're body will force you to do it later.
2.    Look at your form on lighter sets to determine what exactly is going wrong. What's different? Be a problem solver; you may need to pay attention specifically to elbow movement and position on the bench press, or on how different parts of the range of motion feel.
3.    Find an unloaded or lightly loaded way to address the problem you've found. This can include practicing your form with a weight that isn't challenging, or performing a mobilization or therapy-esque exercise to address an imbalance.
4.    Regress your working weights, then work back up with your optimal form.

There's a reason that 'perfect form' is something to shoot for. While perfect form changes from person to person based on a dozen factors, for you it means the technique that allows you to progress without hurting yourself. It means the most efficient form to lift the most weight, the most number of times, over the long haul. This is a hard strategy to implement, as it will slow you down compared to your technique-cheating peers.

Whenever you find yourself making form compromises to add weight, ask yourself if it's strategic or simply an expression of the ego. If your ego is telling you to add weight when your logical brain and technique are telling you not to, you have a big decision to make. Most people ignore this decision, boosting their ego in the short term while ending up with a shattered ego on the exercise bike. Don't be a victim of the ego.

The slow road isn't always the best road, but it is the most reliable strategy in this case. If you squat 20lbs more in five years than you did today, isn't that better than giving up the squat entirely? Regression is a 'check yo-self' moment built into all plans based on sustainability. Like the tortoise and the hare, the sustainable effort will see the most results over time.

Get comfortable with taking a step back, before you're forced to crawl back.

## ACTION

Use your warm-up sets as a measuring stick. Can you perform your exercises perfectly with no weight, or light weights? Are you having trouble with part of the range of motion that was once easy for you? In many cases, simply regressing the exercise to the unloaded version will give you enough diagnostic data, and this will allow you to practice safely. Everyday movements are also good for this; if your mobility changes negatively you may need to look at your exercise technique a little more closely. Pay attention as you put on socks, tie your shoes, reach overhead and perform any other routine movements that should be easy.

Follow the progression models above to ensure you install these regular checkpoints in your program. Additionally, start every workout with bodyweight reps and ensure you keep a full, pain-free range of motion in basic movement patterns before you load anything. If anything seems off or you can't maintain optimal technique at higher weights, it's time to back off the weight and re-approach. This can also mean going to the previous movement in the progression if you're exclusively performing bodyweight work.

Remember; regression is only failure if it's unplanned. Regression that allows you to continue moving forward over time is a win. One step back can earn you two steps forward, which is better than being stuck in the mud.

*The Laws of Strength*

# LAW #6: PLAY THE GAME

For most people, resistance training is a recreational sport. It's a sport rather than an activity because it's inherently competitive and demanding. Though I'm sure most Olympians treat lifting like a sport, most gym-goers do not. This is a problem of perspective and it can seriously hinder your fitness success. Fix the perspective and it can be your secret to dramatic improvements.

For a weightlifter preparing for the Olympics, the sport doesn't end in the gym. These athletes are trying to claw their way into uncharted territory; to do so they need to fire on all cylinders. The sport isn't just lifting...it's a game that includes nutrition, rest and recovery, stress management, and a devotion to the body and mind. This is the perspective you need to achieve your fitness goals.

Too many people want weight loss to be about *one* thing. People will say ridiculous things like, "abs are made in the kitchen", or, "If I train hard enough I can eat whatever I want".

Beyond a certain point the latter may approach the truth, but not many people train that hard. The former statement is just silly, like any other statements that apply arbitrary percentages to diet or exercise for helping you reach a goal. How do you even quantify a percentage split between gym time and the kitchen? Are the units cucumbers or barbells?

There's usually a *most* important answer or factor. This factor is elusive and often requires expert advice to find and change. Even more importantly, this factor will change over time if your body and mind are changing. At one point in your life diet may be the most important consideration for your fat loss, and at another point exercise may trump diet.

Rather than throwing up your hands and ordering a pizza while skipping the gym, you should embrace the fitness lifestyle. The Olympian knows that just working on one factor won't get them to their goal, as they need to do everything optimally. Our stakes are slightly lower in most cases - though fitness can save your life, which is as high as stakes get - but our smaller successes and failures are based on the same scale. Just because we aren't competing in the Olympics doesn't mean we can ignore the major determinants of success.

You need to make your success a game, and you need to play the hell out of it. It isn't a game that's won or lost in the gym, on the treadmill, or in the kitchen. It's a game that's played every second of every day. It's a game that's won or lost based on the sum of your decisions. Every decision you make can bring you closer to your goals or drive you further from them. This process plays out even if you aren't aware of it, so now is the time to realize that you are playing the game whether you want to or not.

Knowing that every moment can bring a small measure of success or failure can bring pressure. Rather than folding under that pressure, treat the game like a game. When you make a good dietary choice, acknowledge your success. Don't celebrate the success with a pizza though, unless that pizza brings you closer to your goals.

Acknowledge that your devotion to your own life, happiness and goals doesn't start and stop based on your attention span. You're succeeding and failing all day every day, you may as well take advantage of your opportunities.

For the novice lifter, this means realizing that staying up all night to binge-watch a TV series might not be the best thing for your recovery. This may mean that you choose to stand at your desk instead of sitting, as sitting tends to tighten your hips and ruins your squats. This could mean that instead of sitting in a recliner while you read, you opt to hit some gentle stretching while reading on the floor instead.

You may have serious lifting goals that are measured in pounds or movement patterns. You could also be more recreational; happy to succeed but it isn't getting you out of bed in the morning. When your goal motivates you, it's enough to shape your lifestyle. If you don't have that motivation just yet, remember that the factors that allow for success in lifting will advance you in many ways in your life.

Focusing 24/7 on what can boost your training efforts means eating better, sleeping better, thinking more clearly and prioritizing, actively de-stressing and recovering as well as being more active generally. Is there anything in your life that wouldn't benefit from these interventions? Lifting success is ultimately determined by your devotion to your body and mind. It's one and the same with honouring yourself and being grateful for the great gifts that you have to work with.

*The Laws of Strength*

Look at your lifting as a sport. Embrace the game that's being played all day whether you pay attention to it or not. Once you see all of your daily opportunities as potential successes or failures, you'll see that the game rewards effort. When you see the rewards, you'll see that the game is worth playing; only then can the big rewards roll in.

## ACTION

Put your lifting under the bright lights. Recognize the inherent value in advancing your lifting practice, and observe as many of the daily factors that bring success as you can. You'll see these factors everywhere, from the choice of parking spots to the use of your leisure time. Support your lifting game in any way you can and you'll automatically improve your life in multiple ways. You don't need to win every moment of every day, but you should accept that most moments contain opportunities to improve yourself or to fall behind.

Embrace the game, and play to win. Apply specific lifting goals to help you with your vision. These goals can be to hit a certain number of bodyweight reps, time challenges, weight challenges, or setting a deadline to hit a certain exercise progression by. Even if you don't need to hit this goal to go to the Olympics, recognize that working for it and attaining it will help you develop in more ways than just 'pounds lifted'.

*The Laws of Strength*

# Law #7: Perseverance and Consistency

Perseverance means to remain steadfast in the face of difficulty and delayed success. This Law probably needs no more explanation than the previous sentence, but I'll elaborate to show you just how important it is. Once you've chosen your path, your goals, your program, and whatever else, you need to chip away at these pursuits consistently. The more time off you take between efforts, the more those efforts disappear into the wispy nothingness of 'could've beens' and 'should've beens'.

Humans tend to enjoy black and white thinking because there is no ambiguity. Life is simpler when you can label something good and bad, and it makes us feel as though we have more control than we really do. The reality is that few things are inherently good or bad, and the circumstances as well as our perspective tends to nudge them one way or another. Not seeing and embracing the grey will limit you dramatically.

Similar to this contrasted thinking is the standard human effort model. I suspect it's a relic from the ancient times when we had to flee from predators then huddle together in basic shelters for warmth. We seem to be built to pursue all-or-nothing efforts, and even our muscles are wired this way. When you fire a muscle fibre, it fires as hard as it can every time even if you are only picking up a paper clip. If the paper clip weighs more, you simply recruit more muscle fibres to help.

We see this all-or-nothing perspective in our friends, colleagues and probably our own health history. When most people decide to lose weight, they begin as completely sedentary people, making poor food choices and generally eating too much. These people aren't accustomed to putting in any effort on themselves.

When they start their effort, they'll begin a ridiculous and restrictive fad diet, start waking up three hours earlier to go to the gym every day for two hour workouts, and also try to hit 10,000 steps per day. While these are all noble efforts, they most often lead to a crash and burn. As you learned in Law #6: Playing the Game, an all-or-nothing effort in your own health is a battle that you will fight on many, many fronts.

The person that can maintain their effort the longest typically has the best results. This is true regardless of the intensity of the effort in many cases, as the above example tends to end in dramatic failure. If the person described above had instead decided to change one meal per day for the better, then two meals, then three, then they decided to add in extra walking, then added the gym over the course of six months, they would be lighter and happier now.

The body adapts to what it's consistently exposed to. It's a basic stimulus-response system. If you eat less today, tomorrow and everyday for the next week, your body will realize that there's no way around losing weight. If you eat less today and binge tomorrow, your body will think, "PHEW! I'm glad that rough patch is over...time to recoup my calories", and you'll eat everything within arms' reach.

117

As you may have guessed, weight loss is largely about calories, regardless of what the unscientific fad diet folk tell you. Eat more, your body adds tissue. Eat fewer calories and your body needs to find energy from your existing tissues. If you want to create a deficit of 2000 calories, you can do it by:

a)   Not eating at all tomorrow. In some circumstances this is used as torture.

OR

b)   Taking 200 calories out of your diet per day, for the next ten days. This is far from torturous, and you won't even notice the difference if you plan it well.

These approaches create the same calorie deficit. However, one of them gives you ten days of better habits and understanding of your choices, as well as ten days of subtle effort that your can body adapt to. The other strategy made you binge for several days following the effort, taught you nothing, ingrained bad habits, and made your body think, "What the hell?".

**Minimum effective doses applied consistently over time will beat bigger efforts applied inconsistently.**

The same will be true in your training. You might not turn into Arnold overnight, and you should be prepared for that disappointment. Chances are, you won't turn into Arnold the next day either. All the while, you'll be putting in effort and changing your life to suit your goals. Are you prepared for that?

They best way to determine if a movement, sport or exercise will injure someone is looking at whether or not they're prepared for it. If you try to set a world record on your first day in the gym, it'll probably wreck you (and not in a good way, either). However, with consistent effort you could potentially achieve some incredible things. If you're prepared in some small way for your efforts, you're safe.

Building muscle and strength will follow the same principle. Give your body a consistent workout to adapt to and it will adapt. Following a similar schedule, performing similar exercises, and increasing the load gradually will reinforce this adaptation. Throwing curveballs at your body just confuses it; you can create hard, random workouts, but your body might not know what to adapt to.

Meatheads and bodybuilders are guilty of this as well. One workout they perform a back squat, then the next leg day focuses on a leg press instead, and the following workout focuses on travelling lunges. There's nothing consistent to adapt to. Choosing to perform a single, primary exercise for each muscle group for at least a few weeks at a time would get them much further ahead, but would require them to abandon their gym-ADHD. Stop 'feeling out' your strategy and start planning it.

*The Laws of Strength*
**Consistent stimuli drive progress. Consistency requires**

**Perseverance.**

When discussing lifting, know that we are always assuming that there's effort involved. You're required to work hard, and anyone that tells you otherwise is lying. Getting stronger, more mobile, and leaner will always require work. That doesn't mean that the journey won't be fun; it's all a matter of perspective.

"In this world, nothing is said to be certain, except death and taxes"
- Benjamin Franklin

This harsh reality might not be worth thinking about on a daily basis, but I add one thing to Ben's statement that you should always keep in mind: hard work. Whatever your day looks like, whatever goals you have, and wherever you're starting from, you need to plan on applying effort consistently.

Consistent, smart work will always require perseverance. By definition, this smart and intelligent work is **work**; you can't snooze your way through it. Smart, intelligent work always plays the long-game: sacrifice your need for instant gratification for a better tomorrow. You will need to persevere in moments that you feel you aren't achieving your goals. You'll need to persevere when you're challenged to complete another set or rep.

You need to maintain your resolve in the face of difficulty and without the comfort of immediate success. If your plan is sound and applied consistently, the results will come.

## ACTION

Follow the Laws in this book. Use my videos and resources to craft a plan, or get help designing an intelligent plan to follow. Persevering through a stupid plan isn't admirable, it's stupid. After you have a smart plan to follow, decide that you'll make a minimal investment in yourself every day. This doesn't need to be a full workout, as a full workout every day might not be the best thing for you.

This investment can be a workout, a walk, a stretching session or massage...it can even be some quiet reflection time or a goal setting session. Plan on being consistent with your efforts, and make yourself comfortable with the fact that your goals won't show up overnight; this is why they're worth chasing in the first place.

Learn to observe and celebrate your small, everyday successes. Even if a workout doesn't go as planned, you can still be happy that you showed up.

Winners don't win because they showed up on the good days, they win because they persevered through all of the days, good and bad. Perseverance isn't just a willpower struggle, it's the ability to keep your mind focused on your vision even when that vision doesn't seem closeby. If you don't need to persevere through anything, you probably aren't working toward anything meaningful. Keep your eyes on the big picture, and win your daily battles.

Erratic, random, and infrequent stimuli won't do much for your progress. Be consistent and clear with your intentions and move your body in the direction you want to go. Small, regular doses applied consistently over time, through thick and thin. This is how you win.

*The Laws of Strength*

*The Laws of Strength*

# LAW #8: PRACTICE, DON'T COMPETE

Whether you want to or not, you're always competing. Though you may consider yourself enlightened and above such things, you probably aren't. It's hard to travel through life without comparing yourself to everything in your frame of reference: what you could do in the past, what you plan to do in the future, and the achievements of peers.

The competition will always be there, especially if you abide by the Laws in this book and learn to implement them to improve your body. You're always competing with your previous rep, set, and session. Keep the fire going and pursue progress as though you really want to beat what you could do yesterday.

As valuable as the competitive spirit can be, competition and practice are exclusive interests. The moment you make your regular lifting sessions into all-out battles for progress is the moment you start sacrificing good habits.

The Westside Barbell Powerlifting method is a great example of both using competition and getting owned by it. The lifters at Westside Barbell in Ohio always have been some of the strongest people on earth. They're savage lifters, and observing the footage of their sessions helps explain why. They have groups of elite lifters; every lifter is surrounded by people that are just as strong, just as motivated, and maybe even more so. Rising to the level of your training partners is inevitable in such a setting, and I think they can attribute much of their success to this culture.

In trying to implement the Westside system, most lifters make the same mistakes. The system asks you to continually work for personal records, and there is pressure in the program to hit PR's regularly. Inevitably, the chase for records will lead lifters to the dark side; they'll throw form, accessory exercises and other important factors under the bus in order to squeeze out a few more pounds on their main lifts.

Your desire for progress is important, but it must be patient, too. You need to treat your process as a practice, not a competition. If you step into the gym every day thinking you need to set a record, you're in trouble. You may get a few records, but you'll probably stop doing the things that led you to those records in the first place.

Treating your lifting like a practice means always *building*. Whether or not you reach new heights or set records, you need to do enough to build yourself for progress down the road. Step into the gym thinking, "I'm going to do whatever I can today to make myself stronger tomorrow, and one year from tomorrow". This consideration will always keep you pointed in the right direction: forward.

Build yourself. Practice your technique with ever increasing weights, ensuring that technique doesn't get sacrificed for short-term gains. Practice your accessory exercises. Practice building your volume and work capacity over time. Practice your recovery methods. Treating all of these essential components as a practice keeps you focused on the right improvements.

127

If you practice heavy back squatting, your form will always be good. It'll be good because you're devoted to improving it and keeping it consistent throughout your workouts and for the duration of your program. If your form is on point consistently, you'll be able to practice with heavier and heavier weights. If you're practicing with heavier weights, you're making your gains.

Too many lifters get drunk with their newfound power and are tempted to continually test their maximal efforts. Most maximal efforts are messy, ugly, and far from perfect. Do this too often and messy, ugly and imperfect will become your new standard.

Treat your training like a practice; it's a pursuit that you want to continually improve at. While at first it seems like this means harder exercises and more weight, it actually means continual improvement. If you aren't practicing well, you can't expect progress to continue for long. Be competitive with yourself, push yourself and compete with others if it helps. Don't sacrifice the more important factors of your lifting success for a little instant gratification.

## Action

Regularly ask for feedback on your lifting technique. Take videos if you can. Take note of how sets, reps and different exercises feel. Note whether the bar is moving quickly or slowly. Note whether you feel you have control of the weight or not. All of these indirect indicators should tell you if your practice is going well.

Start your workout with the right mindset. You're doing this to become better at something specific. Do it poorly and you can't expect much progress. Devote yourself to training well and you'll meet your goals along the way to your next goal. Practice. If you don't feel like you're getting better, take a step back. Watch your videos, read your notes and be objective.

*The Laws of Strength*

*The Laws of Strength*

## LAW #9: THE BODY IS A SINGLE UNIT

We have 640 skeletal muscles, 206 bones and 360 joints. The traditional bodybuilding idea that we can isolate body parts with particular exercises is wrong, and it represents a dangerous game to play.

One can take the simplest exercises - biceps curls, seated knee extensions, and crunches, etc - and realize that the body is a continuous functional system, not a collection of distinct parts. We represent a collection of parts only in anatomical terms, not in functional terms. As you don't live in the pages of an anatomy book, you'd better learn to train for function.

You may reason that the biceps is the only muscle contributing to the 'biceps' curl. You would be wrong. Very wrong. Depending on the angle of the hands, your brachialis and brachioradialis will perform much of the work. The forearm muscles work hard to maintain a neutral wrist. Pec minor can even contribute to your curl strength, especially at the top of the range of motion. This isn't to mention the fact that you need to work to keep your torso upright, you need to provide stability at the shoulder for the biceps to move the arm, and the triceps need to operate as an active brake to prevent excessive elbow flexion velocity. Do you still think you can isolate muscles?

Some exercises are better than others at working specific muscles, but you'd be hard pressed to find an exercise that works one lone muscle. More importantly, you shouldn't try to isolate a muscle outside of clinical efforts. Striving for isolation is usually a one way ticket to creating imbalance.

Bodybuilders may choose to think they're using specific exercises to create balance; but this is in appearance only. Appearance criteria don't hold up to functional needs, they only hold up to the scoring that may win you a bodybuilding competition.

When you take it upon yourself to design, balance and isolate your body in very specific ways, you are trying to outsmart whatever engineering deity designed us in the first place. Good luck with that! The more prevalent outcome is creating a system of imbalances that leaves you misaligned and hurting.

The alternative is to accept and embrace the body as a single, functional unit. This means that you'll no longer use your Push Ups to train your chest, you'll use them to train your chest, core, legs, shoulders, arms and back. In short, pushups are a full body exercise when performed well. Squats, deadlifts, rows, presses, lunges, jumps, running, tumbling and all sports have the same requirement: full body mastery. By embracing this idea you can turn every session into a full body session.

The pushup is a great example of this. Most people will fail because the hips drop: the core fatigues and the change in angle makes the upper body pressing leverage more efficient...because the pressing and core muscles can't keep up with demands.

Rather than strengthening the shoulders in isolation to improve your pushup (as many people do), it's better to contract the quads,

133

glutes, abdominal muscles, back and chest muscles with intensity for the duration of every rep. It'll be exhausting to train this way, but your core won't fail on you. You can't stop yourself from involving all of these muscles, so you might as well make the most of it.

Practice creating as much tension as you can through your body as you perform your familiar exercises. This means squeezing handles and bars as hard as you can, or balling your hand into a fist as you perform bodyweight squats. This means keeping the glutes and abs contracted for the duration of the workout. By creating dramatic, full-body tension we create maximal stability.

Enhancing our stability reduces joint stress, improves the effect of the exercises, and ensures balanced development. Stability is the best way to keep your joints functioning optimally throughout any given range of motion. This stability will keep you safe and ensure that you're always working hard despite the safety.

We don't want to walk around holding maximal tension in all of our tissues. Our everyday life should be without conscious tension. We should seek to minimize undue tension, as is evident from the all-too-common stress-tension in the shoulders. When challenging our body, our range of motion or our movement capacity, tension will keep you safe. In many cases, patients of mine have rid themselves of lingering pain by creating strategic tension in specific movements throughout their day, enhancing their stability and strength.

Creating maximal tension throughout the body may limit the amount of weight you can lift on a given exercise, but it'll also help you maximize the effects of your training. This tension will help you grow stronger over time, whereas a lack of tension could have lead you to plateaus and injuries.

Moreover, full body tension lets you isolate the body on your terms. You can still pick on certain body parts and lacking areas, you simply do it by ensuring your muscles provide all the potential support that they can.

There's a trend emerging in recent research that suggests maximal voluntary muscle contractions - flexing as hard as you can - can lead to muscle growth and strength improvements. While it remains to be seen if these adaptations still exist in those with lots of training experience, you owe it to yourself to use any advantage you can get your hands on.

Lifting this way may hurt your ego and make you sweat. Be prepared to challenge both your body and your ability to focus! This focus will also improve mind-muscle connection, muscle activation, body awareness, and the metabolic fatigue that leads to stronger, more enduring muscles. There are many, many benefits to lifting this way, while the only potential drawback is a knock to the ego.

The body is a singular unit. You can use the entire system to support your efforts, or you can neglect the incredible resources at your disposal. The human body is an incredible piece of engineering. Work the body with compound, multi-joint and full body exercises whenever possible. These movements will support joint health, build structural balance and increase mobility over time.

For the average person, return-on-investment is an important consideration in the gym. It's truly baffling to see a trainer take a client through a 30 minute workout, half of which is spent on arm isolation exercises. If the workout is only 30 minutes long, this is the worst possible use of time. Not only does this approach neglect the bigger, more structurally important and powerful muscles, it also won't lead to much systemic adaptation. If this client had hoped to burn lots of calories or shape the entirety of their body, they're out of luck.

The needless complexity of isolating body parts will get you into trouble. Even if you aren't tempted by your vanity, you'll neglect something, somewhere. Even worse, you won't train your body to act as a functional unit as it needs to in real life. Train movement patterns and functions first, worry about the specific muscles later if you really need to.

## ACTION

Realize that every movement is a full body movement; you can use the rest of the body to help you with the exercise or you can choose not to. Our fascial and connective tissue systems ensure that no corner of our body is separate from the rest of the body: embracing this will help you develop in a balanced way.

Start every set by consciously contracting as many major muscle groups as you can. Focus on the quads, hamstrings, glutes, abdominals, chest and back muscles. You might find that doing this in a standing position brings you closer to perfect posture. Keep these muscles contracted throughout the set, ensuring that you continue your normal breathing. When the set is over, consciously release all this tension and shake your limbs out. This shaking may seem like a basic intervention, but it reliably helps you remove excessive muscular tension.

Remember, we want the tension to help us achieve more in fitness. We don't want conscious tension throughout our day unless we're trying to correct a movement pattern or we don't have time to get to the gym that day.

Choose your exercises with return-on-investment in mind. Squats, lunges, deadlifts, presses, pull-ups and rows are the kings of the exercise world for a reason. These exercises work the entire body at once, even if they train specific parts harder than others. Ensure that the majority of your gymtime is spent on these high-return multi-joint exercises.

Whenever you have the chance to perform an exercise on your feet or standing up, consider doing so. Standing shoulder presses work more of the body than the seated variation. Dumbbell presses work more of the body than machine-based pressing work. Involve as much of your body as possible into every movement, and you'll be in for one hell of a training session.

*The Laws of Strength*

*The Laws of Strength*

# LAW #10: EMBRACE PHYSICAL CULTURE

This is the most important Law in this book and the most important principle for your long term fitness. If you skipped all of the other laws but implemented this one, you would eventually satisfy the requirements of laws one through nine.

Physical Culture is technically a social movement from the 19th Century. Toward the end of the century, diseases of affluence and the changes imposed by improving technology were already beginning to accumulate.

These problems originated from a steep decline in physical requirements of daily life; a problem we face in spades today. The once robust human race was becoming weak thanks to evolving technology...does it still sound like I'm talking about history?

Physical Culture was a diverse and ever-evolving beast. It included recreational sport, weightlifting, strongman competition, dance, gymnastics, calisthenics, and sport borrowed from cultural history like highland games throwing, Indian Clubs, and medicine ball training. The masters and practices of the age are less important than the message the pursuit illustrates.

We've all been born into bodies capable of incredible physical work and feats of strength. Though we have differing personal histories and capabilities, we can all improve and become impressive in our own right. This inheritance is being seriously threatened by modern culture and technological advances.

Kids play differently now. The allure of devices and the internet diminishes the stimulation we once found from playing physically. From an entertainment perspective, there's less need for exploring our physical abilities and experimenting with what we can do.

While we can worry all day about the children, this same problem is occurring for adults ten times as fast. Modern adult life already comes with its own challenges compromising activity; commutes, challenged schedules, stress, sedentary work, and a lack of structure to reinforce the need for activity. It's plain to see that this problem has only accelerated with the advent and prevalence of digital media, handheld devices and so on.

Most people accept these things as the norm, quietly hoping that they won't be debilitated by their life choices. Even if this is the new norm, it isn't right or healthy. Whether or not you consider these things to be conscious choices is irrelevant: you're either choosing physical fitness or physical decline.

The original Physical Culture movement realized these problems and provided alternatives to the new norms. While some weekly gymnastics sessions or recreational sport may have been enough in the 1850's, it isn't enough now. Our non-exercise daily activity is at an all time low. We *need* serious training time and something that will get our butts off the couch outside of training time. Sadly, Pokemon Go probably won't cover your bases either.

Contemporary Physical Culture needs to become our new norm. While we may not need the strength to manually plow fields or hitch wagons, we do need to become fit. We need to stay fit and mobile for as long as possible.

We need fitness on a personal level: imagine what you could achieve if you improved your general fitness. Imagine the pain you could avoid if you improved your fitness. Remember to use fitness in its broad sense here: fitness isn't biceps or abs or body fat percentage, fitness is your ability to act, experience and contribute in meaningful ways throughout your life.

We need fitness interpersonally: to take care of others and to avoid unnecessary care ourselves, as well as to remain a functional member of society, not just social media. We need fitness on a societal level: our bodies heavily influence our minds, our environment and our ability to interact with our world.

Physical Culture means embracing the fact that you were born into the most incredible piece of engineering on this Earth. While this gift has already been bestowed, it's up to you to honour it. It's your privilege to maintain and improve your body so you can experience life to the fullest. Your body is the vessel through which you interact with the world...don't you think a better vessel might improve those interactions?

We are surrounded by so much novelty, so much information and stimulation that we've forgotten the original source of entertainment and development: the body. Your body will transmit every sense to your consciousness, pass along every stimuli and experience to you. The body is literally the vehicle you use to experience the world, and it's directly wired to your mind. The body is the instrument through which we achieve any meaningful action or experience.

Prepare the body to transmit the right messages to your mind: this is the beginning. Improve the organism in all ways and you can both send and receive better messages. Over time, who knows what sensations and messages we may learn to enjoy?

It's too easy to think of exercise, training and activity as work. It's hard for most people to unplug or detach themselves from their problems long enough to really connect the body, mind and the environment. If you can learn to do so, you'll find that movement, physical play and interaction are abundantly interesting and fun on their own, no Netflix or superphone necessary.

It's customary for adults to forget these things, but most of the people reading this book will remember such experiences from childhood. You would swim just for the sake of swimming. You would go for a bike ride and enjoy the exertion, the balancing and the wind rushing past you. You'd jump rope, play hopscotch, tag or try to do a cartwheel just to see if you could. This is the kind of physical exploration we need at every age, in age-appropriate doses.

Physical Culture is about celebrating our gifts by exploring them and enjoying them. It's about being physical...just because we're physical beings, and just because we can. Physical Culture is about building your life around the thing that allows you to experience life: your body. With our physical training we improve the organism as a whole, and our minds become healthier as well. Physical culture means always growing, playing and experimenting physically.

It doesn't matter if you're a Crossfitter, a bodybuilder, a couch potato or an Olympian. The questions remain the same. What can you do? What does it feel like? How can you learn to do more, to see what that feels like?

Embrace the physical nature of our existence. Celebrate it with movement and physical development. Strive to continue growing and expanding in all ways, and pay more attention to the ways that really speak to you. That could be powerlifting or dancing, it doesn't matter.

Develop in all ways, and choose to enjoy the activities that you really love as often as possible. Above all else, learn to love everything physical. You are here, you might as well try it all and make the most of it.

## ACTION

Try new things. Focus on personal and physical growth in all ways. Find things you enjoy that also make you breath hard, things that make you stretch and extend, and things that make you push harder than you could before. Grow in all directions. Try new physical activities just for the fun of it; don't worry about looking stupid or getting embarrassed. These sensations are all part of the game, and you won't be the only newbie that's ever struggled: newbies are supposed to struggle.

Life is interaction with the environment, so get out there and interact. Compete with yourself, compete with others, and play for fun. If you already have a passion or hobby, make sure you grow around it. Pouring yourself into one pursuit can create mastery, but it won't provide you with the full spectrum of experiences we're meant for.

Stand at social events and parties. Go for a walk with your coffee. Get a dog and treat it well. Being physical is part of your everyday life already; the more you embrace it the more you can enjoy it.

We don't live like our ancestors, our predecessors or even our parents. Life is changing for the human race and for us personally all the time. Where you are doesn't matter outside of the context of where you're going, and what you're doing. Embrace all aspects of physical life, and never stop growing.

*The Laws of Strength*

147

# CHAPTER IV

# WHERE TO START

You've got the Laws. You've thought them through and applied them as you've read. Now what? What does the life of a lifter look like when following this system? Where you start will vary slightly depending on what you're starting with, but the necessary foundations are the same.

## For Athletes, Competitors and Experienced Lifters

As an aspiring strength athlete, bodybuilder, or other competitive and experienced trainee, you can begin by immediately changing your existing routine as you read through the book. Each Law will change the way you view individual sets, reps, workouts and even years of training.

Adjust as you go, but also implement the challenges below intended for those starting from scratch. As demeaning as that may sound, many strong, muscled, athletic people I've trained have had bad habits and limitations that they simply avoided confronting. The training years pass, and you may find that the stronger you get at certain lifts the less comfortable you are challenging yourself with your weaknesses. This is a major problem.

I start out all of my assessments with basic movement capacity for this very reason. As the brilliant therapist Gray Cook would say, "Don't layer fitness on top of dysfunction". This essentially means that you found a suboptimal way to move or train, then assumed it was fine and continued to make this pattern stronger. Lifting isn't inherently dangerous, but using lifting to strengthen imbalances rather than correcting them is problematic and common.

As a person or athlete with some training experience, you'll need to continue with some of your former training routine as you implement the Laws. Make sure you test yourself with the beginner progressions below to see exactly where you rank as a physical specimen overall. Your ego may take a bigger beating than your body. In that case, the ego-beating is exactly what you need to continue your progress.

# For Novices

As a complete novice with very little experience, you may not have much ego attached to your physical abilities. This is a great position to start from. Remember: physical development is inherently challenging. It isn't expected to be easy, and having trouble with something is a good thing, not a bad thing. Struggling with an exercise or test means you can learn more from it.

Some of the exercises you'll see in the video progressions will seem intimidating. Some of the challenges below may seem well beyond your capacity. This is a good thing. It doesn't matter where you start out. If you aren't happy with your current fitness level then a little frustration will go a long way. If you could jump right into exercise and master everything in one week you wouldn't need books like this.

You may not consider yourself an athlete. You are. Don't try to argue, as you automatically lose when you try to argue with a book. That would get pretty awkward pretty fast. Everyone is an athlete at a different stage of development. Most of the time competitive athletes will be well ahead of their sedentary counterparts in every physical way. That said, even the elite athletes need to routinely work on basic movements and exercises. The elite and the novice are built of the same material. Train yourself as though you're an athlete; play the game.

*The Laws of Strength*

# For People Experiencing Pain

Pain must be addressed before starting these challenges. Some pains will certainly get better with any movement and exercise. Many pains will get worse, or they're an indicator of something more serious that needs to be considered. Get cleared by your doctor for exercise. If you have pain, have it assessed by a physical therapist that understands and appreciates resistance training.

If you only have pain at particular joint angles and in certain positions, you may be safe to explore the mobility work outlined below. For example, if the start of the squat progression (the top of the range of motion) doesn't hurt anything, you can expand your practice up until the point that you encounter pain. Pain messes with your muscle activation, movement patterns, and it can get in your head. Without a competent coach or therapist present I wouldn't try to work through severe pain.

Get your pain figured out, attack it actively and come back to the exercise testing below when you're ready. If you aren't quite ready for the testing, try using the above principle to expand your capacity. Simply find exercises, activities and movements you can perform without pain, and work more of them into your day.

*The Laws of Strength*

*The Laws of Strength*

# THE CHALLENGES

Implement the tests below to see exactly where you stand. These challenges are meant to be performed in order, starting with mobility and ending with capacity. In this way, we can ensure that you aren't pushing yourself unless you have the basic mobility, stability and strength to support the effort.

These challenges represent the beginning, and something to build upon. This is not an exercise program, nor are these exercises enough to keep you progressing forever if you're consistent. Master the challenges below and add them to your current daily and weekly exercise routines. When you feel ready for more challenges, let me know and I'll gladly write a book of programs and physical methods just for you.

Prior to beginning, a disclaimer: your health is your responsibility. If you require medical clearance or suspect you might need medical clearance before doing any exercise, see your health practitioner. A book is not a substitute for your doctor.

*The Laws of Strength*

# BASIC MOBILITY CHALLENGES

Without basic mobility, you won't be able to do much exercise. Resistance training especially requires you to utilize the full range of motion available to you. Working a muscle with partial movements can be effective, but it isn't the best way to strengthen the body or to maintain your joints and mobility. With adequate mobility, you'll be able to get into lots of fun positions through which you can challenge yourself.

Pain always means a failure in these challenges. If you fail a test, try scaling it back slightly and see if you can perform the movement with less range of motion and no pain. If not, jump ahead to the Basic Stability tests and try those instead. If they also bring pain, you're off to the clinic.

A pass in these tests means you're ready for the next test. Do them in order. Take the easy wins when you can get them, pat yourself on the back, and keep moving.

*The Laws of Strength*

# CHILD'S POSE

The popular yoga pose is a decent diagnostic movement. Though it might not seem like a dramatic mobility test, it's among the most important positions we can asses. If you can perform the full Child's Pose position without pain, it tells us the following:

1.  You can get into full hip and knee flexion, the ultimate requirement for squatting and hinging movements.
2.  You can get into full shoulder flexion, which is important for proper performance of pressing exercises and overhead work.
3.  You can tolerate some flexion in the lower back without pain. This means you probably don't have imminent spinal problems, and that any spinal problems you've had before won't flare up with reasonable spinal flexion.
4.  Holding this position for five deep breaths illustrates that you have read this far and are trying to change your life.

The above criteria aren't always met so easily. If you have pain in this position - it doesn't matter where the pain is - you need to resolve that first. If it's back pain or pain radiating into the legs, you should probably see a therapist, and avoid exercises that put you into spinal flexion for now.

This is why we do this test; if you don't know what flares up a back problem then you're likely to keep flaring it up. With a little rudimentary core work, you can still get into challenging exercise over time but you'll probably need to limit flexion in the lower back as a rule.

**Fail:** Pain. The inability to sit the hips back on top of the lower legs is also a failure. Work these positions and keep your breath deep and consistent.

**Pass:** No pain with the full range of motion described above. Hold for five big breaths and you've earned your first pass.

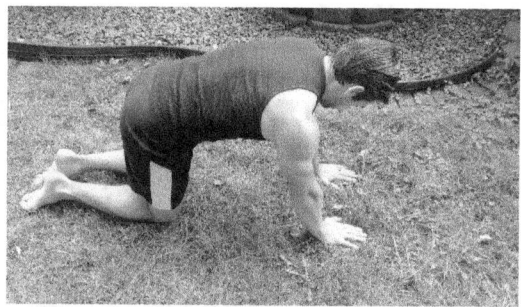

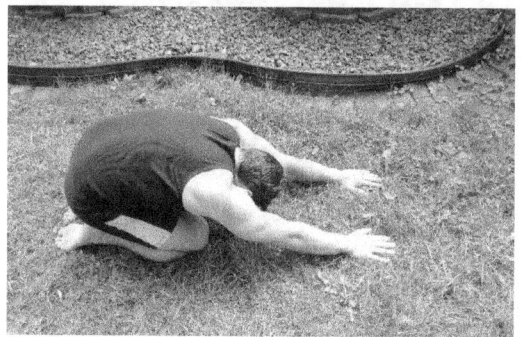

## SLOPPY PUSHUP

This is exactly what it sounds like. Lie on your stomach with your palms flat on the ground beside your shoulders. Keep your hips on the ground as you press your shoulders and upper body off the floor. This should be the ugliest push up you've ever done, and the hips should stay down.

The Sloppy Pushup is another spinal test. This one tells us if you can tolerate spinal extension. Lifters with bad technique will often have trouble with this one, because they load the posterior spine too much. Again, pain here is a fail. Pain in this position tells us that you may need some rehab work, and that you'll likely need to avoid excessive spinal extension in life and exercise for now (this is a good idea MOST of the time anyways).

If you're successful with this exercise, you'll be able to get your elbows fully extended with your hips still on the ground. This tells us that you have adequate spinal and hip extension. Hip extension is one of the golden tickets for long term hip, back and knee health, so make sure you master it here before trying to load it with exercise.

**Fail:** Pain, or the inability to keep the hips down in the top position. Lacking the strength to get to the top position is a fail as well. All of these warrant further work on this exercise, and again you can try the Stability section.

**Pass:** Full range of motion with no pain, hold for a comfortable five breath period.

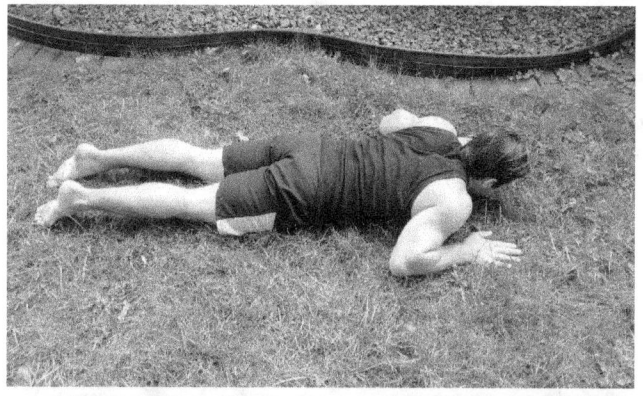

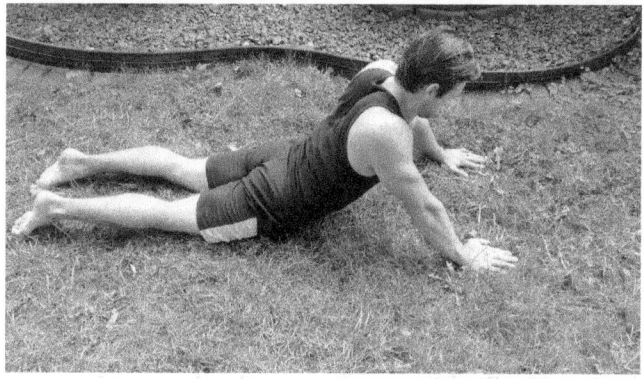

# FORWARD BEND

This is movement is taken from the Functional Movement Screen (FMS). Have yourself assessed by someone trained in FMS if you want a complete diagnostic on your mobility and stability skills. The Forward Bend is also similar to the Hip Hinge movement that's equally important in life and the gym.

Hold a broomstick behind you, with the stick running along the spine from top to bottom. You can use any stick as long as it's straight and unweighted. Hold the stick with one hand behind your head and the other behind your lower back. Keep the stick pressed against the spine and make sure your lower hand never loses contact with your lower back.

When you're comfortable holding this position while standing upright, begin slowly lowering your chest toward the floor **by pushing your butt back**. When the hips move back, the spine is happy and the core is active. Simply bending forward will utilize the spine for support too much; not something we want. Slowly lower as far as you can without the hand leaving the lower back. Keep the knees straight but not locked throughout the movement.

Pause in the bottom position and use a mirror, video, or friend to inform you on how far you moved. We express this range of motion in degrees, with your perfect upright position representing 0 degrees on a 180 degree axis. Bending forward perfectly until your head is level with the hips - which probably won't happen unless you're a current or former dancer/gymnast/contortionist - would give you a score of 90 degrees. Slowly return to the start position.

**Fail:** Pain. If no pain is present, you still fail if you can't reach a 45 degree bend with a straight back. Work this exercise. Practice will help stabilize the movement and loosen the hamstrings, allowing you to get deeper over time. Don't forget to breathe.

**Pass:** You need a pain free 45 degree bend or greater to continue. If you get anything close to 45 degrees, or less than 60 degrees - about halfway between 45 degrees and 90 degrees, visually - you should make this movement part of your daily practice until you improve.

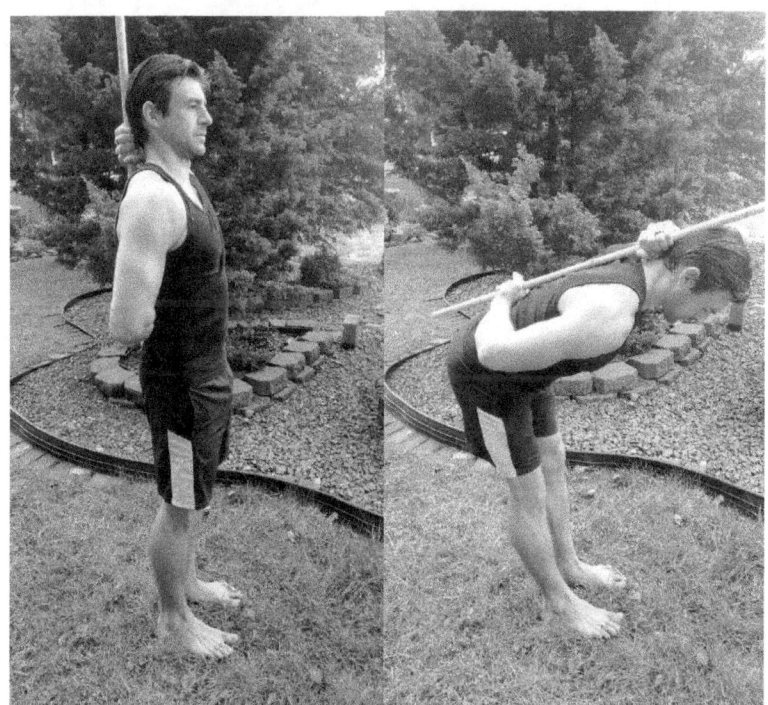

*The Laws of Strength*

# FULL SIDE SPLITS

Just seeing if you're paying attention. You pass this test if you're reading this. If you aren't reading this, you've failed already.

# Basic Stability Challenges

Stability is the quality that allows us to express our mobility in meaningful ways. Those with poor mobility often feel tight all the time, but this tension is usually a lack of stability; they can't actively control their positions in the presence of changing joint angles, load, velocity or unstable conditions. Lots of people stretch and loosen, not many people stabilize.

Lifting will teach you to stabilize your body, but you need to make sure you don't have dramatic imbalances first. Strengthening those imbalances is not the strength training you're interested in. Earn some basic mobility and stability, then you'll be ready to get strong.

# In-Line Lunge

This is another movement variation used in the FMS. In some ways, this movement is more valuable than the squat as a diagnostic. The In-Line Lunge essentially tells us what your single leg strength, stability and mobility are like in a single movement. Single leg strength is important for everyone, as life happens on one leg at a time. Try walking with your feet strapped together and you'll understand this need pretty quickly (this isn't the test, don't actually do this).

Stand on a straight line in the gym or in your home. The line can be the border between two pieces of flooring, the centre of an ab mat...any straight, flat line. Stand with both feet on the line, with one foot in front of you and the other extended behind you. The line should run from the heel through the big toe on each foot, keeping the feet aligned throughout the movement. Between your feet you'll need a space as long as your leg from the knee down.

Now that your footwork is sorted, stand with good posture. Slowly lower your back knee to the floor behind your front foot. Accomplish this movement by squatting with the front leg. Touch the knee down briefly, then hover with the knee about 1-2 inches off the ground. Repeat for the other leg after rising back to the top position.

This is a dynamic test of stability, balance, mobility and strength. It's challenging for most people, couch potatoes and athletes alike. Master this movement and you're ready for some serious exercise.

**Fail:** Yes, pain is a failure. Work the range of motion to see if you can successfully perform partial reps.

**Pass:** Full range of motion with control. Stick the bottom hover position for 20 seconds without falling or taking a break and you're free to proceed. Again, if the duration piece is the problem, use this movement as a training exercise.

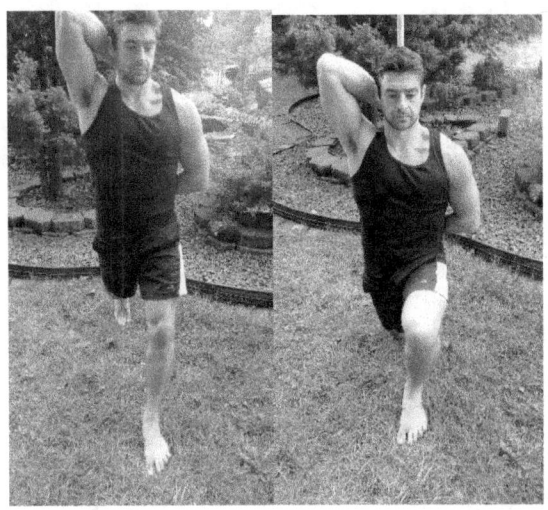

# BIRDDOG

This is a common core exercise. Generally speaking, people tend to think this exercise is easy without realizing they suck at it. It's only really a core exercise if you actively use your core to *resist* movement around the spine. This is an anti-rotation exercise, meaning it challenges your ability to remain stable as gravity tries to twist your spine.

While the primary goal of this exercise is to learn to keep your spine stable in a rotational sense, the spine is also challenged with flexion and extension forces. Most of the time this exercise is performed with a generous amount of spinal rotation, flexion and extension; it's the perfect example of compensation.

To perform this exercise properly, you'll need to move the arms and legs using the shoulder and hip muscles **without** moving the spine. The core muscles must act as they were intended to: they will need to resist pull in every direction to allow the hips and shoulders to do their thing. Do this properly and you'll learn a movement concept that should permeate most of your training sessions. We don't always get into trouble due to immobile joints; often joints move too much.

To perform the exercise, you'll need some soft carpet or an ab mat allowing you to be comfortable in the quadruped position. Rest your weight on your hands and knees with your chest facing the floor. The hands should be placed beneath the shoulders and the knees are placed beneath the hips with the feet resting comfortably on the floor.

Your spine should remain in neutral alignment throughout the exercise, from the top of the head to the tailbone. You'll have some curvature in the spine still; spinal curves are normal. Excessive curves may need correcting. In exercises like this one, it's better to err on the 'flatter' side of this scale. If you need a point of reference, check out your technique in the mirror or lay a broomstick along your spine. The lower back should be able to maintain contact with the broomstick at all times.

Now that you have your basic quadruped position, your primary goal is to keep the spine exactly where it is. Keeping the arms straight, raise one arm directly out in front of you - the upper arm should end up close to your ear - until the hand is at shoulder height in the 'overhead' position.

Simultaneously raise the opposite leg, kicking the knee straight as you lift it until the foot is at hip height. The other limbs remain on the floor for support. Hold the top position briefly, then simultaneously lower the raised limbs and repeat for the other side.

This sounds simple, and many people underestimate the move because they don't understand it. Pretty well everyone has the strength to lift the arm and leg, not everyone has the control to do it without moving the spine. Achieve this unweighted movement without moving your spine and you have a strong, stable core. This movement is all about creating and maintaining stability. When you think about most exercises in the gym, we really don't want your spine moving anywhere as you lift. Therefore, this is a key exercise to master before progressing.

**Fail:** Pain, or the inability to perform the exercise without spinal compensation. If you can't tell, lay the stick on your back so you can feel it out, and take a video if you can. You could also place a small ball or rolly cylinder like a rolling pin or foam roller on your lower back. These things will all let you know if that back is moving right away.

**Pass:** You can demonstrate a nice stiff core and movement  is limited to the moving shoulder and hip. Perform repetitions back and forth between sides with complete control. If you can perform 15 reps per side continuously, you're ready to proceed.

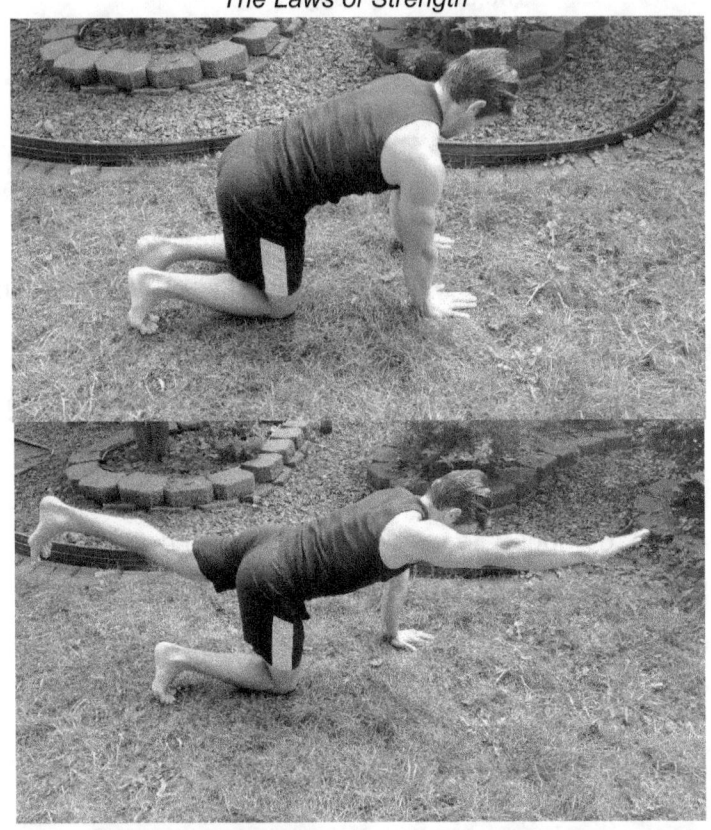

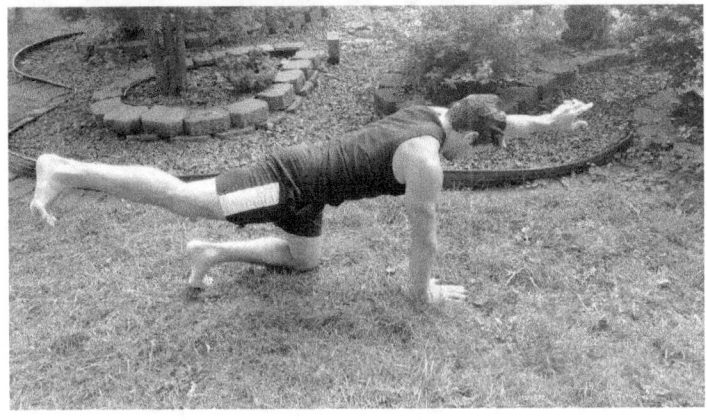

173

# DEADBUG

It's okay to wonder who came up with these exercise names. Just know that BirdDog is better than "Quadruped Opposite Arm and Leg Raise", in my opinion. The Deadbug movement is very similar to what the Birddog tests for, but now the primary challenge is anti-extension of the spine.

Anti-extension is a formal way of saying that your spine is tempted to get into an overextended position, and you need to resist it. This is life, in a nutshell. We carry more weight on the front of our torso, so gravity always pulls us forward slightly. The compensatory result is an over-extension of the lower back to save us from falling on our faces. When this temporary save becomes a long-term strategy, knees get creaky, backs get achy and hips burn.

We're often tempted to default to an over-extended posture in our daily life. This temptation carries over to the gym, where it's commonplace to see people extending their spines as much as possible to get an extra rep on an arm or chest exercise. This is obviously a bad idea. Additionally, no one should enjoy getting owned by gravity. Own the gravitational forces acting on your body. Resist.

To set up the exercise, lie on your back on the floor. Use an ab mat for cushioning if you need it. Touch your lower back to the floor. This will require a slight pelvic tilt, a position that helps engage the deep core muscles. Lift the knees until they're hovering above their respective hips, keeping the knees bent at 90 degrees. Keep the arms straight throughout the exercise and extended with the hands directly over the shoulders. This is your start position. Don't forget the lower back...it needs to keep contact with the floor at all times.

While keeping the lower back touching the floor (I hope these reminders are annoying enough to be effective), slowly lower one leg to the floor as you straighten the knee, allowing the entire posterior leg to come into contact with the floor briefly. Simultaneously lower your opposite-side arm to the floor over your head, keeping the upper arm close to the ear. Pause briefly in the down position, then return to the top and repeat on the opposite side.

As you straighten out diagonally, the spine will be more and more tempted to leave the floor. If that spine comes up, you don't have control. This is a basic bodyweight core drill, if you can't control your spine here you have no business slinging weights around.

**Fail:** Pain. If the lower back leaves the floor, the rep doesn't count. Slow down the range of motion, create lots of core tension by pretending someone is going to step on your stomach, then try again.

**Pass:** Full hip and shoulder range of motion with no limb rotation (your knee may be tempted to move in a semi-circular fashion) on both sides. Repeat for 10 continuous reps per side and you're ready to advance.

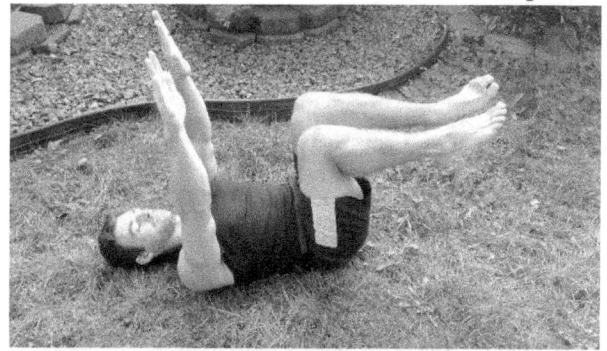

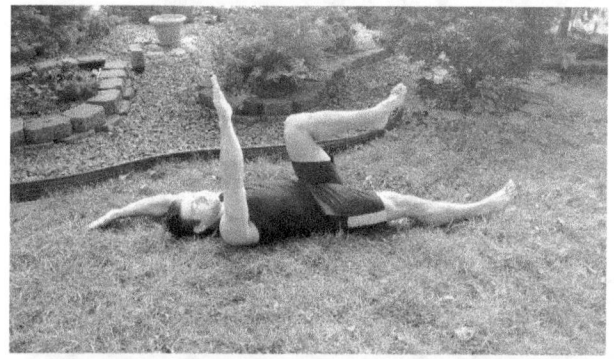

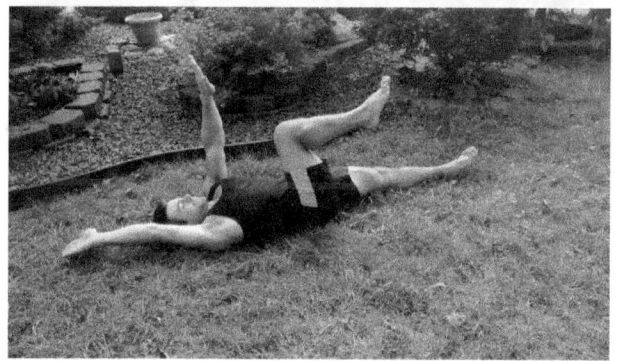

STABILITY SUMMARY

In these three stability tests, you test the core, challenge the spinal, hip, shoulder and knee stabilizers, and mimic the patterns and positions you'll need to use in more challenging exercise down the road. Master these exercises and maintain your mastery: if you've lost the ability to do these well, something has gone wrong.

When you can hit all of these mobility and stability exercises with passing marks, you're ready to test your capacity.

*The Laws of Strength*

# Basic Capacity Challenges

Capacity can be left as vague as it initially sounds. For word count purposes, let's expand the definition anyways. Capacity is the maximum amount that something can contain. In this case, we're referring to how much work you can fit into a given amount of time.

This always implies doing this work correctly, which means that work performed with terrible technique doesn't count towards your capacity at all. Using bad technique only contributes to your capacity to do things with bad technique. If you improve at all with bad technique, those improvements will only last until bad technique breaks you.

Given this vague definition, we can see that capacity is not the same as ability. Ability means you have the skill to execute a task. Capacity expands on ability, requiring you to perform as much work as you can using your ability in a given amount of time. This difference is important; it's often capacity, not ability, that will let you down before an injury.

As you'll know from being alive, life is approximately 50% about resisting fatigue and still getting things done. It really doesn't matter if you have perfect squat technique if you get tired after two reps and your technique gets ugly. You need the capacity to keep that technique in the face of fatigue. Exercise needs to be an interplay between movement quality and capacity. The movement quality always needs to be high, then you need to challenge your ability to do more.

The following tests are basic bodyweight capacity assessments. The movements are basic and the requirements of the tests are basic as well. Though basic, these tests will tell you just how fit you are. Whether you're a novice or an experienced trainee, you need to have the capacity we're testing for here. Without this capacity, future strength, power, mobility and endurance gains will all halt before they need to. Capacity is the workhorse that allows progress to continue across the board.

If the above hasn't quite sunk in just yet, think about capacity as your threshold or rate-limiting-step. Capacity is that threshold beyond which...something will break if we continue. We have a maximum walking, squatting, singing, writing, and smiling capacity. There's always an end limit on what we can do...the idea is to make sure that limit doesn't interfere with what you want to accomplish in life.

Again, approach these tests in the order they appear.

# REVERSE PLANK HOLD

The Reverse Plank is an excellent bodyweight exercise. It lays a solid foundation for upper and lower body pulling exercises, powerful hip extension through a full range of motion, and it works the mobility of the shoulder joint in extension - a position often neglected in the gym.

True to the name, the Reverse Plank essentially picks on the opposite muscles to the Plank, though if you recall from earlier we can never really isolate any muscle. Whereas the Plank uses gravity to pull you into hyper-extension, the Reverse Plank is trying to use gravity to resist hip flexion *and* spinal extension. This means a strong back, hamstrings, glutes and shoulders.

Sit down on the floor with your legs extended out in front of you. Keep the heels touching and the knees extended (no bend, but not fully locked). Rest your hands on the floor just behind and to the outside of your hips, with the palms facing down and the fingers pointing toward the feet. Straighten the elbows and keep them straight.

From this start position, press your shoulder blades as far down as possible. This should lift your hips off the ground. While holding this shoulder position, extend the hips by driving the front of the pelvis toward the ceiling. Extend as far as possible without arching your lower back to move further. Remember, the knees and elbows must remain straight the entire time. Hold the top position, focusing on keeping your pelvis, not your bellybutton, driven toward the ceiling.

Practice a few repetitions to get the movement down then proceed to the challenge. The Reverse Plank capacity challenge is an extension of the Birddog exercise. It challenges very similar muscles in very similar ways, only now we're looking for capacity instead of motor skill.

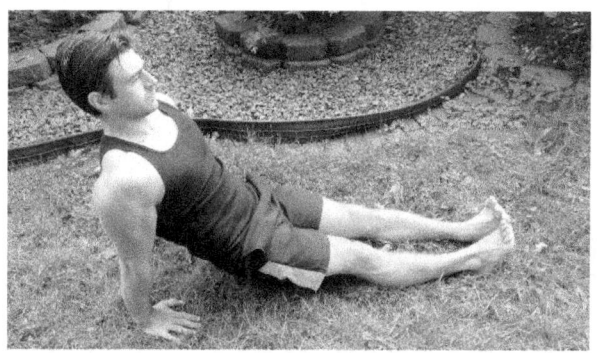

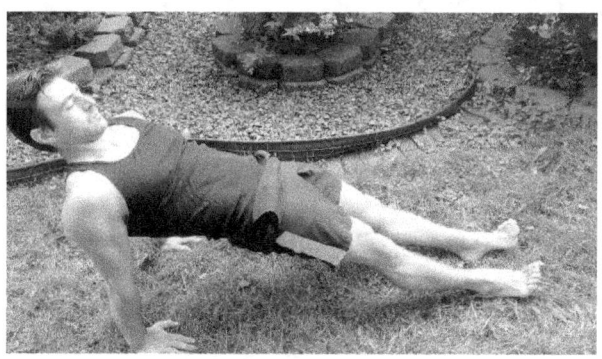

**Challenge:** Perform three sets of 30 second holds in the top position. Rest only 30 seconds between each set. If you don't pass right away, it's okay to move on to the next step and come back to this one after some rest. If your capacity simply isn't there yet, practice the test with whatever duration you can muster, following the same set and rest scheme.

# PLANK HOLD

The Plank is another exercise that's universally panned for being too easy. That said, I don't know that I've ever seen someone perform the exercise correctly before being coached on it. The Plank is an excellent exercise. Perform it well and there are many variations you can try in the future.

The Plank will largely challenge the muscles of the anterior core, the hip flexors, quads and shoulders. This is an extension of the Deadbug: the Plank tests the capacity of the skill you gained practicing Deadbug. Without the ground for feedback, you'll need to be extra diligent to maintain a neutral spinal curve and avoid hyper-extension of the lower back.

Get into position by lying on your stomach on the floor. Now hold for time. Kidding! That probably isn't an appropriate capacity test. Keep your feet pressed together and your knees straight. Arch through the upper back to get your elbows to a resting position on the ground just beneath your shoulders. The hands cannot be allowed to touch each other, as this allows you to cheat and encourages tense shoulders and bad posture.

When you're ready, drive through the balls of your feet and your elbows to lift your hips off the floor. Lift your hips until your body forms a relatively straight line from ankle to shoulder. Use a mirror, friend or video for reference to make sure you're hitting the proper position, then practice getting to this position a few times until you're familiar with what it feels like.

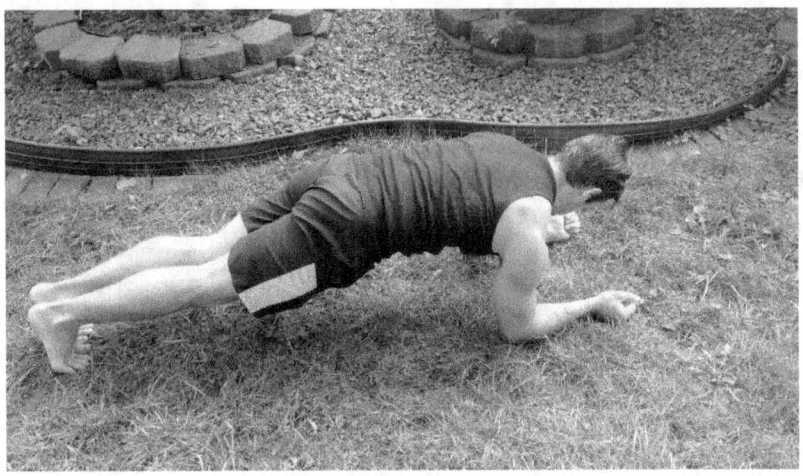

**Challenge:** Hold the top position of the plank with perfect technique for three sets of 30 seconds. Rest only 30 seconds in between sets. Use a timer! No cheating. Letting your form slip or eking out an ugly set only hurts your own interests.

## SQUAT ENDURANCE

Refer to my youtube video on squat technique for all of the technical advice you need to get started.

Once you have a handle on basic technique, you'll need to attain as much range of motion as you can with good form. Start from the top as the video describes, setting up perfect posture. Lower under control by pushing the hips back slightly, then down. The relationship between the ribcage and pelvis shouldn't change throughout the movement, and the spine should remain stable as a result.

One can generally improve their squat range of motion significantly by practicing the movement, strengthening the core and keeping optimal alignment. That said, most of us will encounter skeletal limitations at some point in our squat range of motion. These can't be changed, but they usually don't prevent you from getting a good workout.

Rather than doggedly asking for you to squat until your hips are deeper than your knees (ass-to-grass, or just below parallel), I accept that not everyone will be able to do this with a neutral spine. If you can't do it with a neutral spine then I can't promise that your spine will be safe, and we can't have that.

Try like hell to get your squats as deep as possible with a neutral spine. Stretch, mobilize, get a massage, do corrective exercises, practice your form and get stronger. When you come to that bony barrier, don't ignore it. Injury probabilities increase with loaded spinal movement. Squat as far as you can with a neutral spine and solid control, but go no further. When you find this position, it can be useful to mark it by squatting to a bench, chair or box of that height, touching your butt down on each rep.

After grooving that movement, you'll be ready to test yourself.

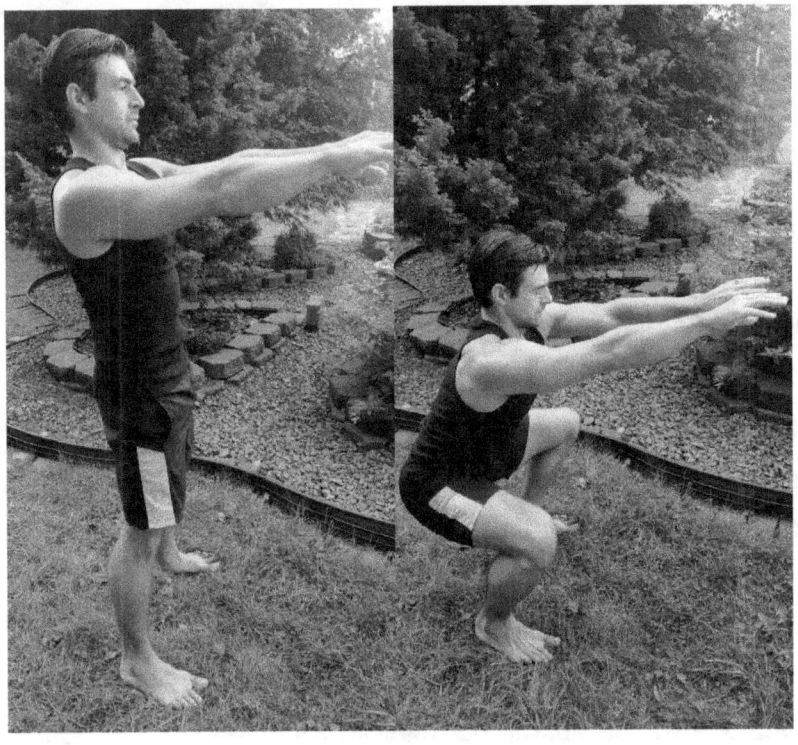

**Challenge:** Perform 300 perfect bodyweight squats for time. Set your range of motion by squatting down until your butt touches a box at the end of your range of motion. Every rep must look the same: touch that box on every rep, and follow the guidelines in the video linked above.

Perform the 300 reps in any way you'd like. You can strategize your sets and reps or simply go until you are forced to take a break. Keep that clock running even when you take your breaks.

This tests your absolute work capacity by making you perform a specific number of reps as quickly as possible. If you complete the challenge, I know you can perform 300 reps of the squat. The time element makes it more interesting and tells us more about your conditioning.

If you complete the reps in less than 10 minutes, you're in great shape and can proceed. If you can do it in less than 15 minutes, you're in decent shape. You can still proceed but you should repeat the challenge again next week, until you can perform the feat in less than 10 minutes.

If it takes you less than 20 minutes to complete the reps, technically you can move. You have some capacity. You need to increase this general capacity before you're prepared for challenges in other exercises. Focus on getting that time down to less than 15 minutes, then less than 10. I'd make this your predominant leg workout until you can do it.

If it takes you more than 20 minutes or you can't do 300 total squats, do what you can. You obviously have room for improvement and this is not a reason to give up. Those with the most improvement to make can make the greatest progress. Perform as many as you can with good technique over the course of 20 minutes. Make this your workout, supplemented with the stability exercises above, until you can hit all 300 in 20 minutes.

One way to track this progress over time is to count your max reps in each 20 minute session from one day to the next. For example, you may only be able to get 30 reps in 20 minutes. Record 30 reps on the calendar. The next day you start the timer again and hit another 30. Repeat the next day, or the day after. See how many days in total it takes you to hit 300 reps. Note how many training sessions it took within those days.

Asking for 300 reps in the squat will be far too easy for some trainees and far too difficult for others. The squat is a fundamental movement pattern for a reason: maintaining our capacity here is important for performance, health, and living an active and safe life. Whether the test is too hard or too easy, do it and maintain the capacity.

*The Laws of Strength*

# PUSHUP ENDURANCE

Refer to my Youtube video primer on Pushup Technique.

The Pushup is a good upper-body correlate of the squat. While many people think of it as a chest and shoulder exercise, it's actually a test of the entire upper body, as well as the core muscles of the hips and the quads.

Practice your technique as outlined in the video mentioned above. Be as strict with yourself as possible. Progress yourself to the point where you can perform strict pushups with your hands on a low bench or with hands on the floor. You can test yourself in either position, just know that performing strict pushups with the hands on the floor is always a goal to work towards, for both men and women.

Strict Pushup technique requires you to touch your nose, chin, or chest to the floor. I require the chest to touch the floor on each rep because it forces you to keep your head in a good position and it makes it nearly impossible to cheat. This is of course an upper-body capacity test, so you'll be performing reps for time. If you don't make chest contact, your rep doesn't count.

As many women I've trained will know, I don't care that you're a woman. I get that training women is different. You have different mobility and stability considerations, hormonal environments and neural profiles.

While these things may be true, there are few major differences in the muscle fibres of men and women. When we compare men and women while taking lean body mass into account, strength differences tend to disappear. You don't need to beat your male counterparts, but you should plan on progressing as though being a woman isn't a drawback. That's a terrible attitude to adopt in the gym.

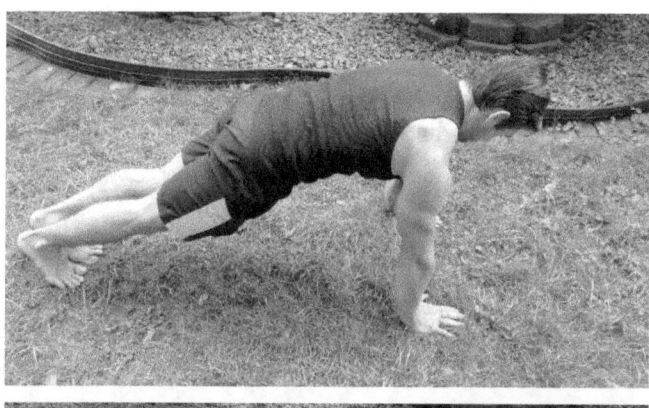

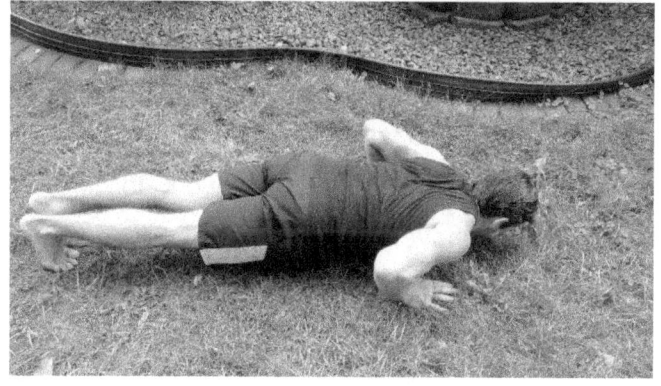

**Challenge:** Perform 150 strict Pushups for time. As with the squats, you can rush, take your time, strategize and plan, as long as you perform all the reps and the clock keeps running. We can use the same time benchmarks as we did in the squat test for this test, as we want upper and lower body capacity to parallel each other as much as possible.

To reiterate: 10 minutes or less means you're a demi-god and you can progress. 15 minutes or less means you're in shape but you should improve your capacity; retest again in one week. 20 minutes or less and you need to get in better shape before challenging yourself further.

If you can't complete all the reps, it takes longer than 20 minutes or you aren't testing on the floor yet, keep at this test by performing 20 minute Pushup workouts. Go for as many reps as you can get (with perfect technique) in 20 minutes, then repeat a few days later. Work up to the 150 total reps, then work on the time component.

As with the above, you can also track how many days and workouts it takes you to get to 150 total pushups. We don't need any ego here: you are where you are and all you can do is work to improve. Give yourself quantifiable challenges and work to beat those challenges over time, just as above.

*The Laws of Strength*

# WALKING

I'm serious. You bought a book about lifting, and you're being challenged with walking? What's this sissy garbage? Before you go full-Rambo on this book, try the challenge. Many big, strong, athletic adults can't stand for half an hour without pain. Seriously.

Your ability to remain on your feet and locomoting for a continuous length of time is important. This is one of the biggest factors in maintaining your quality of life. Internet or no internet, if you can't walk for five minutes without resting your world will be pretty small.

I don't care if you think you're above this test, or if you think it's too basic. Walking is actually a wonderful and complex movement pattern, and you need to maintain it. Even if you're squatting thousands of pounds and flipping cars, you should maintain your ability to walk. The inability to walk briskly for a length of time is a good indicator that you have serious problems lingering just beneath the surface.

This isn't cardio, conditioning, or interval training. This is walking. Practice your ability to locomote from one place to another, and please make sure you've ticked this box before you take on the world.

**Challenge:** Walk briskly and continuously for 30 minutes, three times per week. Don't rest unless you need to. Don't sit down, stop, slow down or break it up into two 15 minute segments. 30 minutes...keep it simple. If you can't walk continuously, if you're uncomfortable, pained or slower than you'd like, work on it. I recommend doing this every week, but you should at least demonstrate you can do it three times per week for one week before moving on.

Complete all of your challenges. Follow the rules, perform them with integrity and objectivity. Check these boxes and you're prepared to push yourself harder toward your goals. Leave the boxes unchecked and you'll have a blemish on your conscience to deal with. Don't complicate things before you need to: there'll be plenty of time for complexity later if you build a good foundation now.

If you can't complete the challenges yet, make these into your primary workouts until you can. Work your mobility, stability, and your basic capacity until you check all of your boxes. It's perfectly safe and practical to perform these tests up to three times each per week until you have them mastered.

*The Laws of Strength*

197

## CHAPTER V

# HOW TO FINISH

The secret to finding the finish line in the fitness race is to accept that this journey takes a lifetime, every time. I'll be the bearer of bad news: you never reach a set-level of fitness that just maintains itself forever. You need to continually work to maintain what you have, and to grow with time.

It's important to walk the fine line between eagerness for progression and satisfaction in your work. Don't be overly positive with yourself if you haven't earned it. Gratuitous positivity only tells your psyche that it's okay to be less than you can be. On the other hand, being so eager for progression that you always hate yourself and look for shortcuts is a dead end street: you'll never be satisfied.

Be happy with yourself for taking the hard road, and the one less travelled. Be satisfied that you're doing something for yourself, regardless of how small or big it is. Be content with your current human-vehicle, but work for upgrades at the same time. Always celebrate that you're walking the path of patience and consistency; the rewards of this path are hidden in plain sight.

Most of all, you need to work. Without ever wanting more, human beings simply wither and die long before their real demise. Don't be one of those. Live the life that you deserve. Feed your body, push it, and reap the benefits for years to come. Put the health and performance of your body before your ego and the need to fit in with the crowd. At the end of the day, you're the only one living in your body and it should fit your needs.

Developing yourself is a task that never ends. This may sound tedious or laborious, but that's continual growth if you take your eyes off the big picture. Continual growth sounds nice, but it isn't particularly compelling until you confront the reality of human existence: if you aren't growing, you're dying. You should seek to grow in many ways, but keep in mind that only physical growth allows you to continue to pursue other paths.

If you need ways to continue developing physically, keep up with Conquest HP online. My website is full of content written to help you reach your goals and find inspiration. The videos on youtube will give you much of the instruction you need to refine your practice.

Remember that these technical instructions will only work with the understanding of the laws that you've just read. Read and reread these Laws until they're a part of you.

Keep growing. Strength doesn't always mean being strong; sometimes it means being weak and seeking to change. Regardless of where you currently stand, recognize the need to move. Standing still gets you nowhere: time will leave the passive behind. Get your feet moving and keep them moving!

EMBRACE AND LIVE THE LAWS. LIFT WELL AND OFTEN!

*The Laws of Strength*

# The Laws, In Stone Tablet Form

1. **Know Thyself** - Be the expert on your own body. Perform your workout            at            your            pace.

2. **Patience** - Record, reflect, be grateful. Progress at the little things and the big things will follow.

3. **Aggression** - Install a switch, then flip the switch. You need to work hard. Make sure the switch doesn't turn off your rational mind.

4. **Progression** - Linear, double, movement progressions...it matters not. Record what you do, push it in measurable increments.

5. **Regression** - Maintain pain free movement throughout your day and in warmup sets. If something doesn't feel right, taking one step back may be the best way to move forward.

6. **Play the Game** - The game isn't just played in the gym. You have chances all day, every day to progress or stall: take advantage of every moment and every factor you can.

7. **Perseverance and Consistency** - Craft a plan that requires a minimum daily investment. Following the plan allows your body to adapt in a coherent direction, all while building good habits and mental strength. Give your body something clear to adapt to, and give it this growth stimulus often.

8. **Practice, Don't Compete** - Become a student of your game, and keep the student mindset through your successes. The practice mindset leads to continual growth, rather than instant gratification.

9. **The Body is a Single Unit** - Train patterns and functions. You can't isolate, so you might as well embrace the interconnectedness of your body. The most interconnected exercises (deads, squats, presses, etc) provide the greatest rewards.

10. **Embrace Physical Culture** - You exist in physical reality - make the most of it. Experiment, exert, and explore your environment. Above all else, enjoy and honour your physical capacity.

*The Laws of Strength*

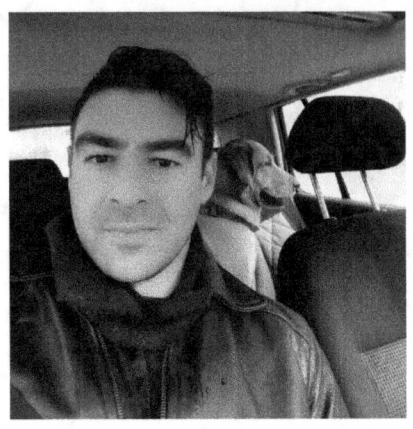

## About the Author

Conor O'Flynn is an Online Fitness Coach, Manual Osteopath, and Writer. He has provided years of manual therapy service in the clinic, during which he has learned some of the intricacies of the human body. He has been practicing as a strength coach since studying kinesiology at Wilfrid Laurier University in Waterloo, Ontario, Canada.

Conor has blended his therapy and Fitness Coaching work into a seamless approach designed to help others reach their goals without destroying the body in the process. Although manual therapy requires a softer touch, Conor believes in being realistic and encourages others to find and express their inner strength.

Conor lives in Sarnia, Ontario, Canada. He writes regularly for his blog (conquesthp.com), frequently shoots videos for his youtube channel (ConquestHP) and is available for contact through either ofthese mediums, as well as on social media (instagram: @ConquestConor).